GUIDELINES
FOR
EXERCISE TESTING
AND
PRESCRIPTION

Senior Editor

W. LARRY KENNEY, Ph.D., FACSM, Professor of Applied Physiology, Noll Physiological Research Center, The Pennsylvania State University, University Park, PA

Associate Editor (Clinical)

REED H. HUMPHREY, Ph.D., P.T., FACSM, Assistant Professor of Physical Therapy, Medical College of Virginia, Virginia Commonwealth University, Richmond, VA

Associate Editor (Fitness)

CEDRIC X. BRYANT, Ph.D., FACSM, Associate Director of Sports Medicine, StairMaster™ Sports/Medical Products, Inc., Kirkland, WA

Authors

DONALD A. MAHLER, M.D., FACSM, Associate Professor of Medicine, Dartmouth-Hitchcock Medical Center, Lebanon, NH

VICTOR F. FROELICHER, M.D., FACSM, Acting Professor of Medicine, Cardiology Section, Stanford University School of Medicine, Palo Alto, CA

NANCY HOUSTON MILLER, R.N., B.S.N., Associate Director, Stanford Cardiovascular Rehabilitation Program, Stanford University Medical Center, Palo Alto, CA

TRACY D. YORK, M.S., Executive Director, The Spa at the Crescent, Dallas, TX

ACSM's GUIDELINES FOR EXERCISE TESTING AND PRESCRIPTION

5th Edition

AMERICAN COLLEGE OF SPORTS MEDICINE

Williams & Wilkins

BALTIMORE•PHILADELPHIA•HONG KONG
LONDON•MUNICH•SYDNEY•TOKYO

A WAVERLY COMPANY
1995

Executive Editor: DONNA BALADO
Developmental Editor: LISA STEAD
Production Coordinator: MARETTE MAGARGLE
Project Editor: ARLENE SHEIR-ALLEN

Williams & Wilkins
Rose Tree Corporate Center
1400 North Providence Rd., Suite 5025
Media, PA 19063-2043 USA

Accurate indications, adverse reactions, and dosage schedules
for drugs are provided in this book, but it is possible they may
change. The reader is urged to review the package information
data of the manufacturers of the medications mentioned.

Printed in the United States of America.

First Edition 1975
Library of Congress Cataloging in Publication Data
Guidelines for exercise testing and prescription / American
    College of Sports Medicine ; {W. Larry Kenney . . .
    [et al.]. — 5th ed.
    p.   cm.
    Includes bibliographical references and index.
    ISBN 0-683-00023-3
    1. Exercise therapy.   2. Heart—Diseases—Patients—
Rehabilitation.   3. Exercise tests.   I. Mahler, Donald A.
II. American College of Sports Medicine.
    [DNLM: 1. Exertion.   2. Exercise Test—standards.
3. Exercise Therapy—standards.   WE 103 G946 1994]
RC684.E9G845   1994
615.8′24—dc20
DNLM/DLC
for Library of Congress   94-40330
                                                 CIP

*The Publishers have made every effort to trace the copyright
holders for borrowed material. If they have inadvertently
overlooked any, they will be pleased to make the necessary
arrangements at the first opportunity*

                              95 96 97 98 99
                          1 2 3 4 5 6 7 8 9 10

Reprints of chapters may be purchased from Williams &
Wilkins in quantities of 100 or more. Call Isabella Wise,
Special Sales Department, (800) 358-3583.

PREFACE

The 5th edition of *ACSM'S Guidelines for Exercise Testing and Prescription* takes yet another major step in the evolution of this manual first published by the American College of Sports Medicine (ACSM) in 1975. As in previous editions of the *Guidelines,* the continued aim of this revision is to present state-of-the-art information in a usable form for both the fitness and clinical exercise professional. Several major changes have been incorporated into this edition, however, which reflect the growing body of knowledge in this area as well as the growing reference needs of the men and women comprising this expanding and diversifying profession. It is hoped that these additions and modifications will expand the utility of this book, bringing it off the office shelf and into the lab coat pocket or onto the desktop in the exercise testing or leadership arena.

One intent of the authors of this revision was to limit the book's focus to exercise testing in its broadest sense and exercise prescription in all of its forms. Toward that goal, some chapters were deleted from the fourth edition (e.g., "Clinical Exercise Physiology"), because these topics are now covered more comprehensively in other ACSM publications. Thus, the 5th edition of the *Guidelines* presents a more narrowed and concise focus on exercise testing and exercise prescription.

At the time of publication of the early editions of the *Guidelines*, companion and complementary publications by ACSM did not exist. There are now several ACSM publications in print or in preparation which complement and expand upon this book. The unique role of the

5th edition of the *Guidelines* is to present easily accessible information relevant to exercise testing and prescription. For more detailed treatment of topics covered in the *Guidelines*, the reader is directed to its companion publication, the *Resource Manual for the Guidelines for Exercise Testing and Prescription (2nd ed.)*. Where minor inconsistencies exist between the *Guidelines* and the *Resource Manual*, the reader is reminded that this is due to differing publication cycles for these two books, and that the former drives the latter. For special populations not covered in the *Guidelines*, the reader is referred to *Exercise Management for Persons with Chronic Diseases and Disabilities*, to be published in 1996. Finally, the *ACSM Fitness Book* provides fitness information and an easy-to-use fitness program designed for use by the apparently healthy adult who wishes to start an exercise program.

A decision was made to include more quantitative data—threshold values, clinical laboratory cutoffs considered "abnormal," normative fitness data—than were included in previous editions. Where appropriate, those values are referenced to reports or publications prepared by other professional organizations. It is not the policy of ACSM to endorse criteria established by one organization over another, but to provide scientifically based, clinically sound guidelines which, in combination with professional judgment, can be used by the exercise professional in decision making.

Also in terms of content, the 5th edition provides expanded information aimed at fitness professionals whose clientele fit into the category of the "apparently healthy adult." Such information is included under the headings of both Exercise Testing (Physical Fitness Testing) and Exercise Prescription. Three healthy "special populations" are covered in greater detail, namely children, pregnant women, and the elderly (Chapter 11). Another area of expanded coverage is testing and prescription for pulmonary patients. Finally, several appendices were added, including a brief ECG interpretation schemata with standard values (Appendix C) and expanded treatment of environmental considerations (Appendix E). Appendix D (Metabolic Calculations) has been completely rewritten to improve its clarity, and Appendix F now presents information about ACSM Certification Programs,[TM] including revised knowledge, skills, and abilities (formerly called Behavioral Objectives and Specific Learning Objectives) underlying each level of certification.

Finally, the most obvious change to the longtime user of the *Guidelines* is the presentation style and format of the book. These changes were made in an effort to increase the utility of the book for the working exercise professional.

This edition has been prepared by a volunteer writing team with representative expertise in physiology, fitness, cardiology, pulmonary medicine, nursing, and physical therapy. It has undergone extensive review by many members of the American College of Sports Medicine. The College and the writing team wish to express their thanks to all those who have contributed ideas, comments, written material, and editorial assistance.

W. Larry Kenney, Ph.D., FACSM
Senior Editor

NOTE BENE

The views and information contained in the 5th edition of *ACSM'S Guidelines for Exercise Testing and Prescription* are provided as *guidelines* as opposed to *standards of practice.* This distinction is an important one, since specific legal connotations may be attached to such terminology. The distinction is also critical inasmuch as it gives the exercise professional the freedom to deviate from these guidelines when necessary and appropriate in the course of exercising independent and prudent judgment. *ACSM'S Guidelines for Exercise Testing and Prescription* presents a framework which the professional may certainly—and in some cases has the obligation to—tailor to individual client or patient needs and alter to meet institutional or legislated requirements.

LIST OF ABBREVIATIONS

AACVPR	American Association of Cardiovascular and Pulmonary Rehabilitation
ACE	angiotensin converting enzyme
ACGIH	American Conference of Governmental Industrial Hygienists
ACOG	American College of Obstetricians and Gynecologists
ACP	American College of Physicians
ACSM	American College of Sports Medicine
ADL	activities of daily living
AHA	American Heart Association
AIHA	American Industrial Hygiene Association
AMA	American Medical Association
AMS	acute mountain sickness
AICD	automatic implantable cardioverter defibrillator
AST	aspartate aminotransferase
AV	atrioventricular
BIA	bioelectrical impedance analysis
BLS	basic life support
BMI	body mass index
BP	blood pressure
BR	breathing reserve
BUN	blood urea nitrogen
C	ceiling (heat stress) limit
CABG(S)	coronary artery bypass graft (surgery)
CAD	coronary artery disease
CHF	congestive heart failure
CHO	carbohydrate
CI	cardiac index
COPD	chronic obstructive pulmonary disease
CPAP	continuous positive airway pressure
CPR	cardiopulmonary resuscitation
CPK	creatine phosphokinase

DBP	diastolic blood pressure
DOMS	delayed onset muscle soreness
ECG	electrocardiogram
EF	ejection fraction
EIB	exercise-induced bronchoconstriction
EIH	exercise-induced hypotension
EL	Exercise Leader$_{SM}$
ERV	expiratory reserve volume
ES	Exercise Specialist$_{SM}$
ETT	Exercise Test Technologist$_{SM}$
FC	functional capacity
FEV$_{1.0}$	forced expiratory volume in one second
F$_I$O$_2$	fraction of inspired oxygen
F$_I$CO$_2$	fraction of inspired carbon dioxide
FN	false negative
FP	false positive
FRV	functional residual volume
FVC	forced vital capacity
GXT	graded exercise test
HAPE	high altitude pulmonary edema
HDL	high density lipoprotein
HFD	Health/Fitness Director®
HFI	Health/Fitness Instructor$_{SM}$
HR	heart rate
HR$_{max}$	maximal heart rate
HR$_{rest}$	resting heart rate
IC	inspiratory capacity
IDDM	insulin-dependent diabetes mellitus
KSAs	knowledge, skills, and abilities
LAD	left axis deviation
LBBB	left bundle branch block
LDH	lactate dehydrogenase
LDL	low density lipoprotein
L-G-L	Lown-Ganong-Levine

LLN	lower limit of normal
LV	left ventricle (left ventricular)
MCHC	mean corpuscular hemoglobin concentration
MET	metabolic equivalent
MI	myocardial infarction
MUGA	multigated acquisition (scan)
MVC	maximal voluntary contraction
MVV	maximal voluntary ventilation
NCEP	National Cholesterol Education Program
NIDDM	noninsulin-dependent diabetes mellitus
NIH	National Institutes of Health
NIOSH	National Institute for Occupational Safety and Health
NYHA	New York Heart Association
P_aO_2	partial pressure of arterial oxygen
PAC	premature atrial contraction
PAR-Q	Physical Activity Readiness Questionnaire
PD	Program Director$_{SM}$
PE_{max}	maximal expiratory pressure
PI_{max}	maximal inspiratory pressure
PNF	proprioceptive neuromuscular facilitation
Po_a	partial pressure of oxygen (ambient)
PTCA	percutaneous transluminal coronary angioplasty
PVC	premature ventricular contraction
PVD	peripheral vacoular disease
R	respiratory exchange ratio
RAD	right axis deviation
RAL	recommended alert limit
RBBB	right bundle branch block
rep	repetition
RIMT	resistive inspiratory muscle training
1-RM	one repetition maximum
RQ	respiratory quotient

RPE	rating of perceived exertion
RV	residual volume
RVG	radionuclide ventriculography
RVH	right ventricular hypertrophy
S_aO_2	% saturation of arterial oxygen
SBP	systolic blood pressure
SPECT	single photon emission computerized tomography
SVT	supraventricular tachycardia
TLC	total lung capacity
TN	true negative
TP	true positive
TPR	total peripheral resistance
TV	tidal volume
VC	vital capacity
$\dot{V}_{CO_2}$	volume of carbon dioxide per minute
$\dot{V}_E$	expired ventilation per minute
$\dot{V}_I$	inspired ventilation per minute
$\dot{V}_{O_2}$	volume of oxygen consumed per minute
$\dot{V}_{O_2max}$	maximal oxygen uptake
$\dot{V}_{O_2peak}$	peak oxygen uptake
VT	ventilatory threshold
WBGT	wet-bulb globe temperature
WHR	waist-to-hip ratio
W-P-W	Wolffe-Parkinson-White
YMCA	Young Men's Christian Association
YWCA	Young Women's Christian Association

CONTENTS

SECTION I.   HEALTH APPRAISAL, RISK
              ASSESSMENT, AND SAFETY
              OF EXERCISE   1

CHAPTER 1.   BENEFITS AND RISKS ASSOCIATED
              WITH EXERCISE   3
              Public Health Perspective   3
              Benefits of Regular Physical
                Activity   4
              Risks Associated with Exercise
                Testing   6
              Risks Associated with Physical
                Activity   8
CHAPTER 2.   HEALTH SCREENING AND RISK
              STRATIFICATION   12
              Health Screening for Physical
                Activity   12
              Risk Stratification   13
              Summary   19

SECTION II.   EXERCISE TESTING   27

CHAPTER 3.   PRE-TEST EVALUATION   29
              Clinical Assessment   29
              Contraindications to Exercise
                Testing   38
              Informed Consent   41
              Patient Instructions   47

CHAPTER 4.   PHYSICAL FITNESS TESTING   49
Purposes of Fitness Testing   50
Basic Principles and Guidelines   51
Body Composition   53
Cardiorespiratory Endurance   63
Muscular Fitness   78
CHAPTER 5.   CLINICAL EXERCISE TESTING   86
Indications and Applications   86
Exercise Test Modalities   91
Exercise Protocols   93
Measurements   94
Post-Exercise Period   100
Indications for Exercise Test
   Termination   100
Radionuclide Exercise Testing   101
Non-Exercise Stress Tests or
   Pharmacological Tests   102
Considerations for Pulmonary
   Patients   102
Summary of Methodology   106
CHAPTER 6.   INTERPRETATION OF TEST DATA   110
Interpretation of Fitness Test Data   110
Graded Exercise Testing as a
   Screening Tool for CAD   112
Interpretation of Responses to Graded
   Exercise Testing   124
Interpretation of Clinical Test Data   130
Predictive Value of Exercise Testing   140
Interpretation of Exercise Tests
   in Pulmonary Patients   146

SECTION III.   EXERCISE PRESCRIPTION   151

CHAPTER 7.   GENERAL PRINCIPLES OF EXERCISE
             PRESCRIPTION   153
Introduction   153
Cardiorespiratory Endurance   156

Caloric Thresholds for Adaptation 166
Rate of Progression 167
Musculoskeletal Flexibility 170
Muscular Fitness 172
Program Supervision 175

CHAPTER 8. EXERCISE PRESCRIPTION FOR CARDIAC PATIENTS 177
Inpatient Programs 178
Outpatient Programs 183
Resistance Training 189
Other Considerations 190

CHAPTER 9. EXERCISE PRESCRIPTION FOR PULMONARY PATIENTS 194
Exercise Prescription 195
Special Considerations 199
Alternative Modes of Exercise Training 201
Program Design and Supervision 203

CHAPTER 10. OTHER CLINICAL CONDITIONS INFLUENCING EXERCISE PRESCRIPTION 206
Hypertension 206
Peripheral Vascular Disease 209
Diabetes Mellitus 213
Obesity 216

CHAPTER 11. EXERCISE TESTING AND PRESCRIPTION FOR CHILDREN, THE ELDERLY, AND PREGNANCY 220
Children 220
The Elderly 228
Pregnancy 235

Appendix A. Common Medications 241
Appendix B. Emergency Management 253
Appendix C. ECG Interpretation and Related Diagnostic Information 263

Appendix D.   Metabolic Calculations   269
Appendix E.   Environmental Considerations   288
Appendix F.   American College of Sports Medicine
              Certifications   297
Index   355

HEALTH APPRAISAL, RISK ASSESSMENT, AND SAFETY OF EXERCISE

chapter 1

BENEFITS AND RISKS ASSOCIATED WITH EXERCISE

PUBLIC HEALTH PERSPECTIVE

An important mission of the American College of Sports Medicine (ACSM) is to promote increased physical activity by the public. While early editions of the *Guidelines for Exercise Testing and Prescription* focused on medically supervised exercise programs, this emphasis has been both amended and expanded to include a broad public health perspective of physical activity and exercise. The need for medically and scientifically sound programs, supervised and conducted by qualified personnel, has not diminished; however, it is increasingly clear that less regimented approaches are needed in community health and activity promotion efforts. The vast majority of physically active adults are not involved in structured, formal exercise programs, nor do they need to be.

BENEFITS OF REGULAR PHYSICAL ACTIVITY

The benefits of physical activity (Table 1–1) are well-established, and emerging studies continue to support an important role for habitual exercise in maintaining overall health and well-being. Persuasive epidemiological and laboratory evidence shows that regular exercise protects against the development and progression of many chronic diseases and is an important component of a healthy lifestyle. Table 1–2 summarizes epidemiological evidence of the efficacy of physical activity in preventing or mitigating the effects of various chronic diseases.[3] Recent studies correlating changes in physical activity in initially sedentary adults with subsequent reductions in mortality have supported the hypothesis that regular activity increases longevity.[1,2] The public health benefits of increasing physical activity within the general population are potentially enormous[4] due to both the prevalence of sedentary lifestyles and the impact of activity on disease risk. Furthermore, data in recent years suggest that the threshold necessary for the health benefits of exercise, such as significantly lowering chronic disease risk, is lower than previously thought. There is a clear inverse relationship between activity and mortality risk across activity categories, and the risk profile indicates that some exercise is better than none, and more exercise—up to a point—is better than less. Thus, public health efforts should be directed toward "getting more people more active more of the time" rather than elevating everyone to an arbitrary fitness or activity level.

TABLE 1–1. BENEFITS OF REGULAR PHYSICAL ACTIVITY*

1. Improvement in Cardiorespiratory Function
   a. Increased maximal oxygen uptake due to both central and peripheral adaptations
   b. Lower myocardial oxygen cost for a given absolute submaximal intensity
   c. Lower heart rate and blood pressure at a given submaximal intensity
   d. Increased exercise threshold for the accumulation of lactate in the blood
   e. Increased exercise threshold for the onset of disease symptoms (e.g., angina pectoris)
2. Reduction in Coronary Artery Disease Risk Factors
   a. (Modestly) reduced resting systolic and diastolic pressures in hypertensives
   b. Increased serum high density lipoprotein (HDL) cholesterol and decreased serum triglycerides
   c. Reduced body fatness
   d. Reduced insulin needs, improved glucose tolerance
3. Decreased Mortality and Morbidity
   a. Primary prevention
      Lower activity and/or fitness levels are associated with higher death rates from coronary artery disease (CAD)
   b. Secondary prevention
      1. Few randomized exercise studies have had a sufficient number of patients and duration to demonstrate the protective effects of exercise; however, most randomized trials report a positive effect of exercise on longevity
      2. Meta-analyses (pooled data across studies) involving post-MI patients provide supportive evidence that a comprehensive cardiac rehabilitation program can reduce premature cardiovascular mortality but probably not nonfatal events
4. Other Postulated Benefits
   a. Decreased anxiety and depression
   b. Enhanced feelings of well-being
   c. Enhanced performance of work, recreational, and sport activities

*Adapted from Reference 4.

TABLE 1–2. SUMMARY OF RESULTS OF STUDIES INVESTIGATING THE RELATIONSHIP BETWEEN PHYSICAL ACTIVITY OR PHYSICAL FITNESS AND INCIDENCES OF SELECTED CHRONIC DISEASES*

Disease or Condition	Number of Studies	Trends across Activity or Fitness Categories and Strength of Evidence
All-cause mortality	***	↓↓↓
Coronary artery disease	***	↓↓↓
Hypertension	**	↓↓
Obesity	***	↓↓
Stroke	**	↓
Peripheral vascular disease	*	→
Cancer		
Colon	***	↓↓
Rectal	***	→
Stomach	*	→
Breast	*	↓
Prostate	**	↓
Lung	*	↓
Pancreatic	*	→
Non-insulin dependent diabetes	*	↓↓
Osteoarthritis	*	→
Osteoporosis	**	↓↓

*Few studies, probably <5; **approximately 5–10 studies; ***>10 studies.
→No apparent difference in disease rates across activity or fitness categories; ↓ some evidence of reduced disease rates across activity or fitness categories; ↓↓ good evidence of reduced disease rates across activity or fitness categories, control of potential confounders, good methods, some evidence of biological mechanisms; ↓↓↓ excellent evidence of reduced disease rates across activity or fitness categories, good control of potential confounders, excellent methods, extensive evidence of biological mechanisms, relationship is considered causal.
*Reprinted with permission from Reference 1.

RISKS ASSOCIATED WITH EXERCISE TESTING

Clinical exercise testing is a relatively safe procedure. Retrospective data from more than 2,000 clinical exercise testing facilities (hospitals and physician offices), in which more than 500,000 tests were performed, have shown a death rate of approximately 0.5 per 10,000 exercise tests and a myocardial infarction (MI) rate of 3.6 per 10,000.[5] A Swedish prospective study (50,000 tests) reported a mortality rate of 0.4 per 10,000, as well as 1.4 MIs and 5.2 hospital admissions per 10,000.[6] In more than 70,000 maximal exercise tests in one preventive medicine clinic there have been no deaths, and only six major medical complications (e.g., MI, ventricular fibrillation, arrhythmias requiring medical treatment, asystole, or stroke).[7]

Surveys evaluating the risks of exercise testing suffer from a lack of uniformity (i.e., they often include both diagnostic and fitness testing, a number of different approaches and philosophies to testing, and a multitude of test modalities and protocols). In addition, they include a wide variety of healthy and diseased populations. It is not possible with the currently available data to stratify risk by population or testing method. The data, however, do suggest that the rate of complications during exercise testing is higher in populations undergoing diagnostic testing, compared with persons being tested as part of a preventive medical examination. The following general statements can be made regarding the safety of maximal graded exercise testing (GXT):

- The risk of death during or immediately after an exercise test is ≤ 0.01%.
- The risk of MI during or immediately after an exercise test is ≤ 0.04%.
- The risk of a complication requiring hospitalization (including MIs) is approximately 0.1%.

The risks associated with submaximal physical fitness testing appear to be even lower. The submaximal cycle ergometer test described in Chapter 5 has been administered to approximately 130,000 adults (ages 18 to 65 years) over the past decade in several worksite health promotion programs and in community health and fitness centers. Pretest screening and exercise testing were performed by nurses or ACSM Certified Exercise Test Technologist$_{SM}$. There have been no deaths or serious medical complications associated with this submaximal fitness testing. The Canadian Aerobic Fitness Test has been used around the world over the past 14 years by an estimated 1 million people. No complications other than minor muscle injuries and isolated episodes of syncope have been reported.[8] Thus, submaximal physical fitness testing appears to have an extremely low risk when accompanied by appropriate pretest screening such as the Physical Activity Readiness Questionnaire (PAR-Q; see Chapter 2) and can be administered safely by qualified personnel in nonmedical settings.

RISKS ASSOCIATED WITH PHYSICAL ACTIVITY

While regular physical activity increases the risk of both musculoskeletal injury and life-threatening cardiovascular events such as cardiac arrest, the incidence is low. Studies of exercise by apparently healthy adults report an acute event rate of 1 per 187,500 person-hours of exercise[7] and a death rate for male joggers of 1 per 396,000 man-hours of jogging.[9] The incidence of cardiac arrest while jogging is approximately 1 episode per year for every 18,000 healthy men,[10] but appears to be lower for men with higher levels of habitual physical activity. This suggests that while the risk of sudden cardiac death is increased during vigorous exercise, this risk is lower among those habitually active. There are no scientifically based studies reporting the incidence of exercise-related cardiac events among women.

The major cause of cardiovascular complications during exercise is coronary artery disease (CAD), and research suggests that the majority of individuals who die during vigorous exercise have one or more CAD risk factors.[9] For patients involved in cardiac rehabilitation programs, an event rate of 1 per 112,000 patient-hours, a myocardial infarction rate of 1 per 300,000 patient-hours, and a mortality rate of 1 per 790,000 patient-hours of exercise have been reported.[11] A more recent report suggests that during medically supervised cardiac rehabilitation exercise programs, the risk of death in the United States is approximately 1 per every 60,000 participant-hours.[12] At this rate, a rehabilitation program with 95 patients exercising 3 hours per week could expect 1 sudden cardiac death every 4 years. In general, the risk is lowest among healthy young adults and non-smoking women, greater for those with CAD risk factors, and highest for those with established cardiac disease. The overall absolute risk in the general population is low, especially when weighed against the health benefits of exercise.

EXERCISE POLICIES AND SAFETY

Lack of uniformity in guidelines and policies for exercise testing and participation has led to much discussion and concern among exercise program personnel. Issues of primary concern include who should be tested, physician attendance during the test, use of maximal versus submaximal testing, and how to classify individuals into risk groups before and after testing.

No matter how rigid or conservative guidelines and policies might be, there is no way to completely eliminate the risk of a serious event during exercise testing or exercise participation. Some data are available to estimate the likelihood of such an event, but clinical and legal judgment, as well as common sense, must be used to make policy decisions involving safety of participants.

Routine diagnostic exercise testing in apparently healthy individuals has limited value.[13] Fitness testing as a screening tool appears to have similar test properties (sensitivity, specificity, and predictive accuracy) as other screening tests, e.g., cholesterol and blood pressure screening. The positive predictive accuracy for all such tests is low (<10%) and the rate of false-positive outcomes is high.[14] Exercise testing is performed in many settings for nondiagnostic purposes, such as worksite health promotion programs, YMCAs and YWCAs, health clubs, and other community exercise programs. This testing tends to be functional [in many cases the electrocardiogram (ECG) is not monitored] and is aimed at assessment of physical fitness, providing a basis for exercise prescription, or monitoring progress in an exercise program. ACSM believes that this type of exercise testing is appropriate for fitness appraisal in conjunction with appropriate screening and when performed by qualified personnel. Such testing programs may be useful in educating participants about exercise and physical fitness and in helping to motivate sedentary individuals to exercise.

REFERENCES

1. Blair SN: 1993 C.H. McCloy Research Lecture: Physical activity, physical fitness, and health. *Res Quart Exerc Sport* *64*:365–376, 1993.
2. Paffenbarger RS, Hyde PH, Wing AL, Lee I-M, Jung DL and Kampert JB: The association of changes in physical-activity level and other lifestyle characteristics with mortality among men. *N Engl J Med 328*:538–545, 1993.
3. Huhn RP: Cardiac rehabilitation in the cost containment environment. *Cardiopulm Phys Ther J 4*:4–8, 1993.

4. Hahn RA, Teutsch SM, Paffenbarger RS and Marks JS: Excess deaths from nine chronic diseases in the United States, 1986. *J Am Med Assoc 264*:2654–2659, 1990.

5. Stuart RJ and Ellestad MH: National survey of exercise stress testing facilities. *Chest 77*:94–97, 1980.

6. Atterhog J-H, Jonsson B and Samuelsson R: A prospective study of complication rates. *Am Heart J 98*:572–579, 1979.

7. Gibbons LW, Blair SN, Kohl HW and Cooper KH: The safety of maximal exercise testing. *Circulation 80*:846–852, 1989.

8. Shephard RJ: Can we identify those for whom exercise is hazardous? *Sports Med 1*:75–86, 1984.

9. Thompson PD, Funk EJ, Carleton RA and Sturner WQ: The incidence of death during jogging in Rhode Island from 1975 through 1980. *J Am Med Assoc 247*:2535–2538, 1982.

10. Siscovick DS, Weiss NS, Fletcher RH and Lasky T: The incidence of primary cardiac arrest during vigorous exercise. *N Engl J Med 311*:874–877, 1984.

11. Van Camp SP and Peterson RA: Cardiovascular complications of outpatient cardiac rehabilitation programs. *J Am Med Assoc 256*:1160–1163, 1986.

12. Haskell WL: The efficacy and safety of exercise programs in cardiac rehabilitation. *Med Sci Sports Exerc 26*:815–823, 1994.

13. American College of Cardiology/American Heart Association. Special report: Guidelines for exercise testing. *Circulation 74*:653A–667A, 1986.

14. Blair SN, Kohl HW and Barlow CE: Cardiovascular fitness and cardiovascular disease. In *Cardiovascular Responses to Exercise*. Edited by GF Fletcher. Mt. Kisco, NY: Futura Publ. Co., 1994.

chapter 2

HEALTH SCREENING AND RISK STRATIFICATION

HEALTH SCREENING FOR PHYSICAL ACTIVITY

To optimize safety during exercise testing and participation, and to permit the development of a sound and effective exercise prescription, initial screening of participants relative to important health factors is necessary for both the apparently healthy and those with chronic disease. The purposes of the preparticipation health screening include:

- Identification and exclusion of individuals with medical contraindications to exercise.
- Identification of individuals with disease symptoms and risk factors for disease development who should receive medical evaluation before starting an exercise program.
- Identification of persons with clinically significant disease considerations who should participate in a medically supervised exercise program.
- Identification of individuals with other special needs.

It is essential that health screening procedures be valid, cost-effective, and time-efficient. Procedures range from self-administered questionnaires to sophisticated diagnostic tests. The Physical Activity Readiness Questionnaire (PAR-Q)[1] has been recommended as a minimal standard for entry into low-to-moderate intensity exercise programs (Fig. 2–1). The PAR-Q was designed to identify the small number of adults for whom physical activity might be inappropriate or those who should have medical advice concerning the most suitable type of activity.[2]

It is further recommended that persons interested in participation in organized exercise programs be evaluated for signs or symptoms suggestive of cardiopulmonary disease (Table 2–1) and for coronary artery disease risk factors (Table 2–2).

RISK STRATIFICATION

Once some initial level of screening has occurred, it is often desirable to stratify individuals considered for exercise testing or who plan to increase their physical activity on the basis of likelihood of untoward events. This becomes increasingly important as disease prevalence increases in the population under consideration. Participants and patients can be initially classified into three risk strata (Table 2–3) for triage and preliminary decision making.

For cardiac populations, patients may be further stratified using published criteria. Two such risk stratifications [American College of Physicians (ACP)[3] and American Association of Cardiovascular and Pulmonary Rehabilitation (AACVPR)[4]] are presented in Table 2–4. While differing slightly, the two risk stratification paradigms are similar, and either may be used.

Physical Activity Readiness
Questionnaire - PAR-Q
(revised 1994)

PAR - Q & YOU

(A Questionnaire for People Aged 15 to 69)

Regular physical activity is fun and healthy, and increasingly more people are starting to become more active every day. Being more active is very safe for most people. However, some people should check with their doctor before they start becoming much more physically active.

If you are planning to become much more physically active than you are now, start by answering the seven questions in the box below. If you are between the ages of 15 and 69, the PAR-Q will tell you if you should check with your doctor before you start. If you are over 69 years of age, and you are not used to being very active, check with your doctor.

Common sense is your best guide when you answer these questions. Please read the questions carefully and answer each one honestly: check YES or NO.

YES	NO	
☐	☐	1. Has your doctor ever said that you have a heart condition <u>and</u> that you should only do physical activity recommended by a doctor?
☐	☐	2. Do you feel pain in your chest when you do physical activity?
☐	☐	3. In the past month, have you had chest pain when you were not doing physical activity?
☐	☐	4. Do you lose your balance because of dizziness or do you ever lose consciousness?
☐	☐	5. Do you have a bone or joint problem that could be made worse by a change in your physical activity?
☐	☐	6. Is your doctor currently prescribing drugs (for example, water pills) for your blood pressure or heart condition?
☐	☐	7. Do you know of <u>any other reason</u> why you should not do physical activity?

FIG. 2-1. PAR-Q form. Reprinted with permission from Reference 7.

Continued on Next Page

YES to one or more questions

Talk with your doctor by phone or in person BEFORE you start becoming much more physically active or BEFORE you have a fitness appraisal. Tell your doctor about the PAR-Q and which questions you answered YES.

- You may be able to do any activity you want—as long as you start slowly and build up gradually. Or, you may need to restrict your activities to those which are safe for you. Talk with your doctor about the kinds of activities you wish to participate in and follow his/her advice.
- Find out which community programs are safe and helpful for you.

DELAY BECOMING MUCH MORE ACTIVE:

- if you are not feeling well because of a temporary illness such as a cold or a fever—wait until you feel better; or
- if you are or may be pregnant—talk to your doctor before you start becoming more active.

Please note: If your health changes so that you then answer YES to any of the above questions, tell your fitness or health professional. Ask whether you should change your physical activity plan.

NO to all questions

If you answered NO honestly to all PAR-Q questions, you can be reasonably sure that you can:

- start becoming much more physically active—begin slowly and build up gradually. This is the safest and easiest way to go.
- take part in a fitness appraisal—this is an excellent way to determine your basic fitness so that you can plan the best way for you to live actively.

If you answered

Informed Use of the PAR-Q: The Canadian Society for Exercise Physiology, Health Canada, and their agents assume no liability for persons who undertake physical activity, and if in doubt after completing this questionnaire, consult your doctor prior to physical activity.

You are encouraged to copy the PAR-Q but only if you use the entire form

Continued on Next Page

FIG. 2–1. Continued

NOTE: If the PAR-Q is being given to a person before he or she participates in a physical activity program or a fitness appraisal, this section may be used for legal or administrative purposes.

I have read, understood and completed this questionnaire. Any questions I had were answered to my full satisfaction.

NAME _____

SIGNATURE _____ DATE _____

SIGNATURE OF PARENT _____ WITNESS _____
or GUARDIAN (for participants under the age of majority)

© Canadian Society for Exercise Physiology
Société canadienne de physiologie de l'exercice

Supported by: Health   Santé
                  Canada   Canada

FIG. 2–1. Continued

TABLE 2–1. MAJOR SYMPTOMS OR SIGNS SUGGESTIVE
OF CARDIOPULMONARY DISEASE*

1. Pain, discomfort (or other anginal equivalent) in the chest, neck, jaw, arms, or other areas that may be ischemic in nature
2. Shortness of breath at rest or with mild exertion
3. Dizziness or syncope
4. Orthopnea or paroxysmal nocturnal dyspnea
5. Ankle edema
6. Palpitations or tachycardia
7. Intermittent claudication
8. Known heart murmur
9. Unusual fatigue or shortness of breath with usual activities

*These symptoms must be interpreted in the clinical context in which they appear, since they are not all specific for cardiopulmonary or metabolic disease.

The American Heart Association (AHA) has developed a more extensive classification system for cardiac patients[5] (Table 2–5). This table is useful in several ways. First, the AHA provides guidelines for participant/patient monitoring and supervision and for activity restriction. Second, reference is made to the functional classification of the patients according to the well known New York Heart Association (NYHA) criteria,[6] which in turn is used by the American Medical Association (AMA) in its *Guides to the Evaluation of Permanent Impairment.*[7] Whenever such systems are used, results of exercise testing may dictate reclassification of individuals prior to exercise training.

When gas exchange parameters are measured, these values can be used for assessment of functional impairment.[8] Table 2–6 presents a system based on measured $\dot{V}O_{2max}$, ventilatory threshold (VT), and cardiac index (CI, cardiac output normalized for body surface area).

No set of guidelines for exercise testing and participation can cover all situations. Local circumstances and policies vary and specific program procedures are also

TABLE 2–2. CORONARY ARTERY DISEASE RISK FACTORS*

Positive Risk Factors	Defining Criteria
1. Age	Men > 45 years; women > 55 or premature menopause without estrogen replacement therapy
2. Family history	MI or sudden death before 55 years of age in father or other male first-degree relative, or before 65 years of age in mother or other female first-degree relative
3. Current cigarette smoking	
4. Hypertension	Blood pressure ≥ 140/90 mm Hg, confirmed by measurements on at least 2 separate occasions, or on antihypertensive medication
5. Hypercholesterolemia	Total serum cholesterol > 200 mg/dL (5.2 mmol/L) (if lipoprotein profile is unavailable) or HDL < 35 mg/dL (0.9 mmol/L)
6. Diabetes mellitus	Persons with insulin dependent diabetes mellitus (IDDM) who are > 30 years of age, or have had IDDM for > 15 years, and persons with noninsulin dependent diabetes mellitus (NIDDM) who are > 35 years of age should be classified as patients with disease
7. Sedentary lifestyle/ physical inactivity	Persons comprising the least active 25% of the population, as defined by the combination of sedentary jobs involving sitting for a large part of the day and no regular exercise or active recreational pursuits

Negative Risk Factor	Comments
1. High serum HDL cholesterol	> 60 mg/dL (1.6 mmol/L)

Notes: (1) It is common to sum risk factors in making clinical judgments. If HDL is high, subtract one risk factor from the sum of positive risk factors, since high HDL decreases CAD risk; (2) Obesity is not listed as an independent positive risk factor because its effects are exerted through other risk factors (e.g., hypertension, hyperlipidemia, diabetes). Obesity should be considered as an independent target for intervention.

*Adapted in part from *J Am Med Assoc 269*:3015–3023, 1993.

TABLE 2–3. INITIAL RISK STRATIFICATION

1. Apparently healthy	Individuals who are asymptomatic and apparently healthy with no more than one major coronary risk factor (see Table 2–2)
2. Increased risk	Individuals who have signs or symptoms suggestive of possible cardiopulmonary (see Table 2–1) or metabolic disease and/or two or more major coronary risk factors (see Table 2–2)
3. Known disease	Individuals with known cardiac, pulmonary, or metabolic disease

properly diverse. To provide some general guidance on exercise program issues, ACSM suggests the recommendations presented in Table 2–7 for determining when a diagnostic medical examination and exercise test are appropriate and when physician coverage is recommended. In all situations where exercise testing is performed, site personnel should be trained and certified in CPR.

SUMMARY

The health benefits of regular exercise are confirmed by numerous research studies, and broad recommendations to the public to be physically active are appropriate. A potentially negative impact on physical activity participation may arise from suggesting that exercise is dangerous, or insisting that all sedentary persons receive medical clearance prior to becoming more active. The financial cost and limited availability of qualified health personnel and facilities in relation to the large volume of medical evaluations and exercise testing required to comply with overly cautious recommendations make such recommen-

TABLE 2–4. AMERICAN COLLEGE OF PHYSICIANS (ACP) AND AMERICAN ASSOCIATION OF CARDIOVASCULAR AND PULMONARY REHABILITATION (AACVPR) RISK STRATIFICATION CRITERIA FOR CARDIAC PATIENTS*

ACP	AACVPR
LOW RISK	
Uncomplicated MI or CABG	Uncomplicated MI, CABG, angioplasty, or atherectomy
Functional capacity ≥ 8 METS 3 weeks after clinical event	Functional capacity ≥ 6 METS 3 or more weeks after clinical event
No ischemia, left ventricular dysfunction or complex arrhythmias	No resting or exercise-induced myocardial ischemia manifested as angina and/or ST segment displacement
	No resting or exercise-induced complex arrhythmias
Asymptomatic at rest with exercise capacity adequate for most vocational and recreational activities	No significant left ventricular dysfunction (EF ≥ 50%)
INTERMEDIATE (MODERATE) RISK	
Functional capacity < 8 METS 3 weeks after clinical event	Functional capacity < 5–6 METS 3 or more weeks after clinical event
Shock or CHF during recent MI (< 6 months)	Mild to moderately depressed left ventricular function (EF 31 to 49%)
Failure to comply with exercise prescription	Failure to comply with exercise prescription
Inability to self-monitor heart rate	
Exercise-induced ST-segment depression < 2 mm	Exercise-induced ST-segment depression of 1–2 mm or reversible ischemic defects (echocardiography or nuclear radiography)

Continued on Next Page

TABLE 2–4. *Continued*

ACP	AACVPR
HIGH RISK	
Severely depressed LV function (EF < 30%)	Severely depressed LV function (EF ≤ 30%)
Resting complex ventricular arrhythmias (low grade IV or V)	Complex ventricular arrhythmias at rest or appearing or increasing with exercise
PVCs appearing or increasing with exercise	
Exertional hypotension (≥ 15 mm Hg decrease in systolic pressure during exercise)	Decrease in systolic blood pressure of > 15 mm Hg during exercise or failure to rise consistent with exercise workloads
Recent MI (<6 months) complicated by serious ventricular arrhythmias	MI complicated by CHF, cardiogenic shock, and/or complex ventricular arrhythmias
Exercise-induced ST-segment depression > 2 mm	Patients with severe CAD and marked (> 2 mm) exercise-induced ST-segment depression
Survivor of cardiac arrest	Survivor of cardiac arrest

Abbreviations: CABG = coronary artery bypass graft; MET = metabolic equivalent; EF = ejection fraction; CHF = congestive heart failure; LV = left ventricular; PVC = premature ventricular contraction.

*Adapted from References 3 and 4.

dations inadvisable. Virtually all sedentary individuals can begin a moderate exercise program safely; and if large numbers adopt a more active way of life, the public health will be enhanced. The degree of medical supervision of exercise tests varies appropriately from physician-supervised tests to situations in which there may be no physician present. The degree of physician supervision may vary with local policies and circumstances, the health status of the patient, and the experience of the lab-

TABLE 2–5. AMERICAN HEART ASSOCIATION (AHA) RISK STRATIFICATION CRITERIA*

Class A: Apparently healthy
- Individuals < 40 years of age without symptoms or known presence of heart disease, no major risk factors, and a normal exercise test.

Supervision or monitoring required: none

Class B: Documented, stable cardiovascular disease with low risk of cardiac events during vigorous exercise, but slightly greater than for apparently healthy individuals
- CAD (including myocardial infarction, CABG, PTCA, angina pectoris, abnormal exercise test, and abnormal coronary angiograms) whose condition is stable and who have all of the following clinical characteristics:
  1. NYHA Class 1 or 2
  2. Exercise capacity 5–6 METS
  3. No evidence of heart failure
  4. Free of ischemia or angina at rest or on the exercise test at or below 6 METS
  5. Appropriate rise in systolic blood pressure during exercise
  6. No sequential premature ventricular contractions
  7. Ability to self-monitor exercise intensity
- Valvular heart disease
- Congenital heart disease
- Cardiomyopathy
- Exercise test abnormalities that do not meet the criteria outlined in Class C or D below

Supervision or monitoring required: Medical supervision and ECG and blood pressure monitoring only during prescribed sessions; nonmedical supervision of other exercise sessions if the patient can self-monitor activity

Class C: Documented, stable cardiovascular disease with low risk for vigorous exercise but unable to self-regulate activity or to understand recommended activity levels
- Includes individuals with the disease states and clinical characteristics outlined above in Class B but without the ability to self-regulate activity

Supervision or monitoring required: Medical supervision and ECG and blood pressure monitoring only during prescribed sessions; nonmedical supervision of other exercise sessions to help regulate activity

Continued on Next Page

TABLE 2–5. *Continued*

Class D: Those at moderate to high risk for cardiac complications during exercise

- CAD with:
  1. Two or more previous MIs
  2. NYHA Class 3 or greater
  3. Exercise capacity < 6 METS, ischemic horizontal or downsloping ST depression $\geq$ 4.0 mm, or angina during exercise
  4. Fall in systolic blood pressure with exercise
  5. A medical problem that the physician believes may be life-threatening
  6. Previous episode of primary cardiac arrest
  7. Ventricular tachycardia at a workload < 6 METS
- Cardiomyopathy
- Valvular heart disease
- Exercise test abnormalities not directly related to ischemia
- Previous episode of ventricular fibrillation or cardiac arrest that did not occur in the presence of an acute ischemic event or cardiac procedure
- Patients with complex ventricular arrhythmias that are uncontrolled at mild to moderate work intensities with medication
- Individuals with 3-vessel or left main disease
- Individuals with low ejection fractions (< 30%)

Supervision or monitoring: Continuous ECG monitoring during rehabilitation sessions until safety is established, usually 6 to 12 sessions or more; medical supervision during all rehabilitation sessions until safety is established.

Class E: Unstable disease with activity restriction

- Unstable angina
- Heart failure that is not compensated
- Uncontrollable arrhythmias
- Severe and symptomatic aortic stenosis
- Other conditions that could be aggravated by exercise

No activity is recommended for conditioning purposes.

Attention should be directed to treating the patient and restoring him or her to Class D or higher. Daily activities must be prescribed based on individual assessment by the patient's personal physician.

*Adapted from Reference 5.

TABLE 2–6. FUNCTIONAL CLASSIFICATION OF PATIENTS BASED ON GAS EXCHANGE AND CARDIAC INDEX CRITERIA*

Severity of Impairment	Functional Class	$\dot{V}o_{2max}$ (ml·kg^{-1}·min^{-1})	VT	maximal CI (l·min^{-1}·m^{-2})
None to Mild	A	>20	>14	>8
Mild to Moderate	B	16–20	11–14	6–8
Moderate to Severe	C	10–15	8–10	4–5
Severe	D	<10	<8	<4

*Reprinted with permission from Reference 8.

oratory staff. The appropriate protocol is based on the age, health status, and physical activity level of the person to be tested. Whenever possible, testing should be performed by ACSM-certified personnel, since those certification programs evaluate knowledge, skills, and abilities directly related to exercise testing.

REFERENCES

1. Thomas S, Reading, J and Shephard RJ: Revision of the Physical Activity Readiness Questionnaire (PAR-Q). *Can J Sport Sci* 17:338–345, 1992 (based on the British Columbia Department of Health, PAR-Q Validation Report, 1975).
2. Shephard RJ, Thomas S, and Weller I: The Canadian Home Fitness Test. *Sports Med 11*:358, 1991.
3. Health and Policy Committee, American College of Physicians, Cardiac rehabilitation services. *Ann Int Med 15*:671–673, 1988.
4. American Association of Cardiovascular and Pulmonary Rehabilitation. *Guidelines for Cardiac Rehabilitation Programs, 2nd ed.* Human Kinetics Books, Champaign, IL 1994.
5. Fletcher GA, et al: AHA Medical Scientific Statement. Exercise Standards: A Statement for Health Professionals from the American Heart Association. *Circulation 82*:2286–2322, 1990.

TABLE 2-7. ACSM RECOMMENDATIONS FOR (A) MEDICAL EXAMINATION AND EXERCISE TESTING PRIOR TO PARTICIPATION AND (B) PHYSICIAN SUPERVISION OF EXERCISE TESTS

A. Medical examination and clinical exercise test recommended prior to:

	Apparently Healthy		Increased Risk*		Known Disease†
	Younger‡	Older	No Symptoms	Symptoms	
Moderate exercise§	No‖	No	No	Yes	Yes
Vigorous exercise¶	No	Yes#	Yes	Yes	Yes

B. Physician supervision recommended during exercise test:

	Apparently Healthy		Increased Risk*		Known Disease†
	Younger‡	Older	No Symptoms	Symptoms	
Submaximal testing	No‖	No	No	Yes	Yes
Maximal testing	No	Yes#	Yes	Yes	Yes

*Persons with two or more risk factors (see Table 2-2) or one or more signs or symptoms (see Table 2-1).

†Persons with known cardiac, pulmonary, or metabolic disease.

‡Younger implies ≤ 40 years for men, ≤ 50 years for women.

§Moderate exercise as defined by an intensity of 40% to 60% $\dot{V}_{O_2max}$; if intensity is uncertain, moderate exercise may alternately be defined as an intensity well within the individual's current capacity, one which can be comfortably sustained for a prolonged period of time, that is, 60 minutes, which has a gradual initiation and progression, and is generally noncompetitive.

‖A "No" response means that an item is deemed "not necessary." The "No" response does not mean that the item should not be done.

¶Vigorous exercise is defined by an exercise intensity > 60% $\dot{V}_{O_2max}$; if intensity is uncertain, moderate exercise may alternately be defined as exercise intense enough to represent a substantial cardiorespiratory challenge or if it results in fatigue within 20 minutes. For physician supervision, this suggests that a physician is in close proximity and readily available should there be an emergent need.

#A "Yes" response means that an item is recommended.

6. Criteria Committee, NYHA. *Diseases of the Heart and Blood Vessels: Nomenclature and Criteria for Diagnosis, 6th ed.* Little Brown, and Co., NY, 1964.
7. American Medical Association: *Guides to the Evaluation of Permanent Impairment.* AMA, Chicago, 1990.
8. Weber KT, Janicki JS, and McElroy PA: Determination of aerobic capacity and the severity of chronic cardiac and circulatory failure. *Circulation 76*(suppl. VI):40–46, 1987.

section II

EXERCISE TESTING

chapter 3

PRE-TEST EVALUATION

CLINICAL ASSESSMENT

The extent to which medical evaluation is necessary prior to exercise testing depends on the assessment of risk as determined from the procedures outlined in Chapters 1 and 2. The medical evaluation may include a medical history, physical examination, and evaluation of blood pressure, serum cholesterol and lipoproteins, additional blood variables, and pulmonary function. This chapter presents information related to each of these evaluative procedures. The goal is neither to be totally inclusive nor to supplant more specific references on each subject, but rather to provide a concise set of guidelines for pre-exercise test decision making.

MEDICAL HISTORY, PHYSICAL EXAMINATION, AND LABORATORY TESTS

The pretest medical history should be thorough and include both remote and recent past history. Components of a patient history are presented in Table 3–1.

TABLE 3–1. COMPONENTS OF THE MEDICAL HISTORY

1. **Medical diagnoses**—cardiovascular disease including myocardial infarction, angioplasty, cardiac surgery, coronary artery disease, angina, and hypertension; pulmonary disease including asthma, emphysema, and bronchitis; cerebrovascular disease, including stroke; diabetes; peripheral vascular disease; anemia; phlebitis or emboli; cancer; pregnancy; osteoporosis; emotional disorders; eating disorders
2. **Previous physical examination findings**—murmurs, clicks, other abnormal heart sounds, other unusual cardiac findings, abnormal blood lipids and lipoproteins, high blood pressure, or edema
3. **History of symptoms**—discomfort (pressure, tingling, pain, heaviness, burning, numbness) in the chest, jaw, neck, or arms; lightheadedness, dizziness, or fainting; shortness of breath; rapid heart beats or palpitations, especially if associated with physical activity, eating a large meal, emotional upset, or exposure to cold
4. **Recent illness, hospitalization, or surgical procedures**
5. **Orthopedic problems**, including arthritis; joint swelling; any condition that would make ambulation or use of certain test modalities difficult
6. **Medication use, drug allergies**
7. **Other habits,** including caffeine, alcohol, tobacco, or recreational drug use
8. **Exercise history**—information on habitual level of activity: type of exercise, frequency, duration, and intensity
9. **Work history** with emphasis on current or expected physical demands, noting upper and lower extremity requirements
10. **Family history** of cardiac, pulmonary, or metabolic disease, stroke, sudden death

For some, but not all types of testing, a preliminary physical examination should be performed by the attending physician or other qualified personnel prior to testing (see Table 2–7). Essential components of a physical examination specific to subsequent exercise testing are found in Table 3–2.

Certain special tests may be done for risk stratification purposes, to further clarify the need for and extent of

TABLE 3–2. COMPONENTS OF THE PHYSICAL EXAMINATION

1. Body weight; in some instances, determination of body composition (percent body fat) may also be desirable
2. Pulse rate and regularity
3. Resting blood pressure, supine and standing
4. Auscultation of the lungs with specific attention to uniformity of breath sounds in all areas (absence of rales, wheezes, and other breathing sounds)
5. Palpation of the cardiac apical impulse
6. Auscultation of the heart with specific attention to murmurs, gallops, clicks, and rubs
7. Palpation and auscultation of carotid, abdominal, and femoral arteries
8. Palpation and inspection of lower extremities for edema and presence of arterial pulses
9. Absence or presence of xanthoma and xanthelasma
10. Follow-up examination related to orthopedic or other medical conditions which would limit exercise testing
11. Tests of neurological function, including reflexes

intervention, assess response to treatment, or determine the need for additional assessment. Such evaluations, however, are not absolutely necessary for safe conduct of an exercise test if history and physical examination findings are satisfactory. Based on clinical status or risk assessment, Table 3–3 identifies recommended laboratory tests by level of risk and clinical status.

BLOOD PRESSURE

Measurement of resting blood pressure (BP) is an integral component of the pretest evaluation. Decisions should be based on the average of two or more BP readings measured during each of two or more visits following an initial screening.[1] Optimal BP with respect to cardiovascular risk is systolic pressure < 120 mm Hg and diastolic BP < 80 mm Hg.[1] In addition to high BP readings, unusually

TABLE 3–3. RECOMMENDED LABORATORY TESTS BY LEVEL OF RISK AND CLINICAL ASSESSMENT

1. Apparently healthy or high risk individuals
   - Total serum cholesterol; other lipoproteins as indicated (see Figure 3–1)
   - Fasting blood glucose, if indicated by family history or symptoms
2. Patients with coronary disease
   - Above tests plus pertinent previous cardiovascular laboratory tests (e.g., resting 12-lead ECG, coronary angiography, radionuclide or echocardiography studies, previous exercise tests)
   - Chest x-ray, if congestive heart failure is present or suspected
   - Comprehensive blood chemistry panel and complete blood count as indicated by history and physical examination (see Table 3–7)
3. Patients with pulmonary disease
   - Chest x-ray
   - Pulmonary function tests (see Tables 3–8 and 3–9)
   - Other specialized pulmonary studies (e.g., oximetry or blood gas analysis)

low readings should also be evaluated for clinical significance. Table 3–4 provides blood pressure information for the purposes of classification of hypertension, as recommended by the Joint Committee on Detection, Evaluation, and Treatment of High Blood Pressure.[1]

CHOLESTEROL AND LIPOPROTEINS

An increased blood cholesterol level, specifically a high concentration of low density lipoprotein (LDL) cholesterol or a low concentration of high density lipoproteins (HDL) cholesterol, increases the risk of coronary artery disease (CAD). Conversely, lowering total cholesterol and LDL cholesterol reduces the risk. The following material, part of the National Cholesterol Education Program

TABLE 3–4. CLASSIFICATION OF BLOOD PRESSURE FOR ADULTS AGED 18 YEARS AND OLDER*†

Systolic (mm Hg)	Diastolic (mm Hg)	Category
<130	<85	Normal
130–139	85–89	High normal
140–159	90–99	Mild (Stage 1) hypertension
160–179	100–109	Moderate (Stage 2) hypertension
180–209	110–119	Severe (Stage 3) hypertension
≥210	≥120	Very severe (Stage 4) hypertension

†Not taking antihypertensive medication and not acutely ill. When systolic and diastolic pressures fall into different categories, the higher category should be selected.

*Reprinted with permission from Reference 1.

(NCEP),[2] can be used to classify individuals based on cholesterol and lipoprotein concentrations (Table 3–5), determine what type and when follow-up testing is desired (Figure 3–1), and provide information upon which treatment decisions can be made.

The link between triglycerides and CAD is complex. Elevated serum triglycerides are positively correlated with CAD, but they lose their ability to predict CAD when other lipid risk factors are added to the model. Elevated serum triglycerides may indicate the need to evaluate the presence of alcohol abuse, diabetes, steroid use, dietary patterns, and obesity. The NCEP has provided a separate classification scheme for serum triglycerides (Table 3–6). Increased physical activity, coupled with other forms of nonpharmacological therapy (e.g., weight loss in obese patients, alcohol restriction), is recommended for all patients with elevated serum triglycerides.[2] Drug therapies may be indicated if there are associated atherogenic dyslipidemias or very high serum triglyceride levels.

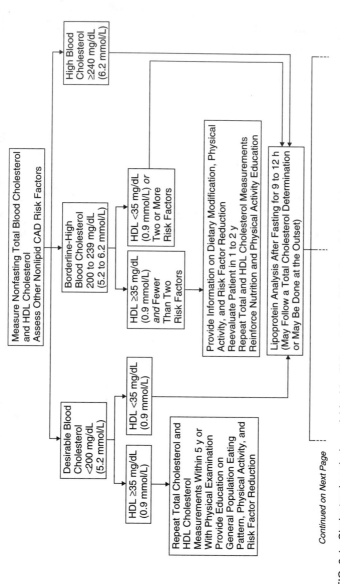

Continued on Next Page

FIG. 3-1. Cholesterol analysis useful for identifying at-risk individuals and determining appropriate follow-up regarding evaluation and therapy.

FIG. 3-1. Continued

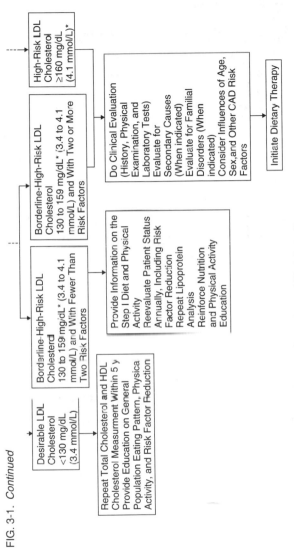

Desirable LDL Cholesterol <130 mg/dL (3.4 mmol/L)	Borderline-High-Risk LDL Cholesterol 130 to 159 mg/dL* (3.4 to 4.1 mmol/L) and With Fewer Than Two Risk Factors	Borderline-High-Risk LDL Cholesterol 130 to 159 mg/dL* (3.4 to 4.1 mmol/L) and With Two or More Risk Factors	High-Risk LDL Cholesterol ≥160 mg/dL (4.1 mmol/L)*
Repeat Total Cholesterol and HDL Cholesterol Measurement Within 5 y Provide Education on General Population Eating Pattern, Physical Activity, and Risk Factor Reduction	Provide Information on the Step I Diet and Physical Activity Reevaluate Patient Status Annually, Including Risk Factor Reduction Repeat Lipoprotein Analysis Reinforce Nutrition and Physical Activity Education	Do Clinical Evaluation (History, Physical Examination, and Laboratory Tests) Evaluate for Secondary Causes (When indicated) Evaluate for Familial Disorders (When indicated) Consider Influences of Age, Sex, and Other CAD Risk Factors	
		Initiate Dietary Therapy	

*On the basis of the average of two determinations. If the first two LDL-cholesterol test results differ by more than 30 mg/dL (0.7 mmol/L), a third test result should be obtained within 1 to 8 weeks and the average value of the three tests used.

TABLE 3–5. CLASSIFICATION OF TOTAL SERUM CHOLESTEROL AND SERUM LOW (LDL) AND HIGH DENSITY LIPOPROTEIN (HDL) CHOLESTEROL LEVELS*

Total Cholesterol	Classification
<200 mg/dL (5.2 mmol/L)	Desirable cholesterol
200–239 mg/dL (5.3–6.2 mmol/L)	Borderline high cholesterol
>240 mg/dL (6.2 mmol/L)	High cholesterol

LDL Cholesterol	Classification
<130 mg/dL (3.4 mmol/L)	Desirable LDL cholesterol
130–159 mg/dL (3.4–4.1 mmol/L)	Borderline high LDL cholesterol
≥160 mg/dL (4.1 mmol/L)	High LDL cholesterol

HDL Cholesterol	Classification
<35 mg/dL (0.9 mmol/L)	Low HDL cholesterol

*Reprinted with permission from Reference 2.

TABLE 3–6. CLASSIFICATION OF FASTING SERUM TRIGLYCERIDE LEVELS*

Serum Triglycerides	Classification	Comments
<200 mg/dL (2.3 mmol/L)	Normal	
200–400 mg/dL (2.3–4.5 mmol/L)	Borderline high	Check for accompanying primary or secondary dyslipidemias
400–1,000 mg/dL (4.5–11.3 mmol/L)	High	Check for accompanying primary or secondary dyslipidemias
>1,000 mg/dL (11.3 mmol/L)	Very high	Increased risk for acute pancreatitis

*Reprinted with permission from Reference 2.

BLOOD PROFILE ANALYSES

Multiple analysis blood profiles are commonly performed in clinical exercise programs. Such profiles may provide useful information about an individual's overall health status and ability to exercise and may explain ECG abnormalities. Some caution is advised when comparing blood chemistries from different laboratories, due to varied methods of assaying blood samples. Table 3–7 gives normal ranges for selected blood chemistries, derived from a variety of sources. These should be applied judiciously and not used as finite ranges of normal.

PULMONARY FUNCTION

Pulmonary function assessment via routine spirometry is another test often used, particularly in patients with diagnosed pulmonary disease or who present with a medical

TABLE 3–7. TYPICAL RANGES OF NORMAL VALUES FOR SELECTED BLOOD VARIABLES IN ADULTS

Variable	Men	Gender Neutral	Women
Hemoglobin (g/dL)	13.5–17.5		11.5–15.5
Hematocrit (%)	40–52		36–48
Red cell count (x10^{12}/L)	4.5–6.5		3.9–5.6
Mean cell hemoglobin concentration (MCHC)		30–35 (g/dl)	
White blood cell count		4–11 (x10^9/L)	
Platelet count		150–450 (x10^9/L)	
Fasting glucose		60–114 mg/dL	
Blood urea nitrogen (BUN)		4–24 mg/dL	
Creatinine		0.3–1.4 mg/dL	
BUN/Creatinine ratio		7–27	
Uric acid (mg/dL)	4.0–8.9		2.3–7.8
Sodium		135–150 mEq/L	
Potassium		3.5–5.5 mEq/L	
Chloride		98–110 mEq/L	
Osmolality		278–302 mOsm/kg	
Calcium		8.5–10.5 mg/dL	
Calcium, ion		4.0–5.2 mg/dL	
Phosphorus		2.5–4.5 mg/dL	
Protein, total		6.0–8.5 g/dL	
Albumin		3.0–5.5 g/dL	
Globulin		2.0–4.0 g/dL	
A/G ratio		1.0–2.2	
Iron, total (μg/dL)	40–190		35–180

history or physical examination that warrants assessment of basic lung function. While many spirometric tests are available, the most commonly used include forced vital capacity (FVC), forced expiratory volume in 1 second ($FEV_{1.0}$), $FEV_{1.0}$/FVC ratio, and maximal voluntary ventilation (MVV). Normal values for lung function are based on age, gender, and height. As such, there are no "best" reference equations for predicting normal lung function, and considerable variability exists for commonly used prediction equations. Automated and computerized equipment often arbitrarily selects equations so that obtained test values may be compared with normal values. Table 3–8 provides a commonly used set of prediction equations.[3,4] Even when properly performed, pulmonary function tests must be interpreted with caution due to the degree of subject cooperation necessary to achieve optimal values, and the wide range of interindividual variability in "normal" responses. For this reason, Table 3–8 also gives the "lower limit of normal" (LLN) for each variable. Subtracting this value from that calculated from the equation provides a better basis for determining whether a test result should be further evaluated.

Table 3–9 presents typical effects of obstructive or restrictive pulmonary disease on spirometric and airflow volume measurements. It should be emphasized, however, that pulmonary function test results provide information that is closely related to other clinical data and as such should not be interpreted in isolation.

CONTRAINDICATIONS TO EXERCISE TESTING

There are certain individuals for whom the risks of testing outweigh the potential benefits. It is important in these circumstances to carefully assess the potential

TABLE 3–8. PULMONARY FUNCTION PREDICTION EQUATIONS WITH CORRESPONDING VALUES CONSITUTING THE LOWER LIMITS OF NORMAL (LLN)*

Women	Prediction Equation	LLN
FVC (L)	$= (0.0414 \times \text{Ht, cm}) - (0.0232 \times \text{Age}) - 2.20$	−0.73
$FEV_{1.0}$(L)	$= (0.0268 \times \text{Ht, cm}) - (0.0251 \times \text{Age}) - 0.38$	−0.55
$FEV_{1.0}$/FVC(%)	$= (-0.2145 \times \text{Ht, cm}) - (0.1523 \times \text{Age}) + 124.5$	−11.1
MVV (L/min)	$= 40 \times FEV_{1.0}(L)$	N/A

Men		
FVC (L)	$= (0.0774 \times \text{Ht, cm}) - (0.0212 \times \text{Age}) - 7.75$	−0.84
$FEV_{1.0}$(L)	$= (0.0566 \times \text{Ht, cm}) - (0.0233 \times \text{Age}) - 4.91$	−0.68
$FEV_{1.0}$/FVC (%)	$= (-0.1314 \times \text{Ht, cm}) - (0.1490 \times \text{Age}) + 110.2$	−9.2
MVV (L/min)	$= 40 \times FEV_{1.0}(L)$	N/A

*These equations are valid for white men and women ages 18 to 85; for African-Americans and Asians, multiply the predicted FVC and $FEV_{1.0}$ values by 0.85. The LLN should likewise be multiplied by 0.85. FVC and FEV equations are from Reference 3; the predicted MVV equation is from Reference 4.

TABLE 3–9. TYPICAL EFFECT OF OBSTRUCTIVE AND RESTRICTIVE PULMONARY DISEASE ON SPIROMETRIC VOLUME AND FLOW MEASUREMENTS*

Measurement	Obstructive	Restrictive
Tidal volume (TV)	N or ↑†	N or ↓†
Inspiratory capacity (IC)	N or ↓	N or ↓
Expiratory reserve volume (ERV)	N or ↓	N or ↓
Vital capacity (VC)	N or ↓	↓ or ↓
Forced vital capacity (FVC)	N or ↓	N or ↓
Residual volume (RV)	↑	N or ↓
Functional residual volume (FRV)	↑	N or ↓
Total lung capacity (TLC)	↑	N
Forced expiratory volume in 1 sec (FEV$_{1.0}$)	↓	N or ↑
FEV$_{1.0}$/FVC	↓	N or ↓
Forced expiratory flow rate between 25% and 75% FVC	↓	N or ↓
Maximal voluntary ventilation (MVV)	↓	N or ↓
Peak expiratory flow	↓	N or ↓

*Adapted from Reference 5.
†N = normal; ↓ = decreased; ↑ = increased.

information to be derived and determine that these outweigh the risks. Table 3–10 outlines absolute and relative contraindications to exercise testing. Exercise tests should not be performed by patients with absolute contraindications until those conditions are stabilized. Patients with relative contraindications may be tested only after careful evaluation of the risk-benefit ratio. It should be emphasized, however, that contraindications may not apply in certain specific clinical situations, such as after MI or surgical patients or to determine the need for, or benefit of, drug therapy. Finally, conditions exist that preclude reliable diagnostic ECG information from exercise testing [e.g., left bundle branch block (LBBB)]. The test may still provide useful information on exercise capacity and hemodynamic responses to exercise.

INFORMED CONSENT

Obtaining adequate informed consent from exercise participants is an important ethical and legal consideration prior to exercise testing and participation in a supervised exercise program. While the content and extent of consent forms may vary, it is important that enough information be present in the informed consent process to ensure that the participant knows and understands the purposes and risks associated with the test or exercise program. The consent form should include a statement indicating that the patient has been given an opportunity to ask questions about the procedure and has sufficient information to give informed consent. If the subject to be tested is a minor, a legal guardian or parent must sign the consent form. It is advisable to check with authoritative bodies (hospital risk management, institutional review boards, legal counsel) to determine what is appropriate for an acceptable informed consent process. Sample consent forms are provided in the

TABLE 3–10. CONTRAINDICATIONS TO EXERCISE TESTING

Absolute Contraindications:

1. A recent significant change in the resting ECG suggesting infarction or other acute cardiac event
2. Recent complicated myocardial infarction (unless patient is stable and pain-free)
3. Unstable angina
4. Uncontrolled ventricular arrhythmia
5. Uncontrolled atrial arrhythmia that compromises cardiac function
6. Third degree AV heart block without pacemaker
7. Acute congestive heart failure
8. Severe aortic stenosis
9. Suspected or known dissecting aneurysm
10. Active or suspected myocarditis or pericarditis
11. Thrombophlebitis or intracardiac thrombi
12. Recent systemic or pulmonary embolus
13. Acute infections
14. Significant emotional distress (psychosis)

Relative Contraindications:

1. Resting diastolic blood pressure > 115 mm Hg or resting systolic blood pressure >200 mm Hg
2. Moderate valvular heart disease
3. Known electrolyte abnormalities (hypokalemia, hypomagnesemia)
4. Fixed-rate pacemaker (rarely used)
5. Frequent or complex ventricular ectopy
6. Ventricular aneurysm
7. Uncontrolled metabolic disease (e.g., diabetes, thyrotoxicosis, or myxedema)
8. Chronic infectious disease (e.g., mononucleosis, hepatitis, AIDS)
9. Neuromuscular, musculoskeletal, or rheumatoid disorders that are exacerbated by exercise
10. Advanced or complicated pregnancy

following text. No sample form should be adopted for a specific program unless approved by local legal counsel.

When the test is for purposes other than diagnosis or

(General) Informed Consent for an Exercise Test (Sample)

1. Explanation of the Test
You will perform an exercise test on a cycle ergometer or a motor-driven treadmill. The exercise intensity will begin at a low level and will be advanced in stages depending on your fitness level. We may stop the test at any time because of signs of fatigue or changes in your heart rate, electrocardiogram (ECG), or blood pressure. It is important for you to realize that you may stop when you wish because of feelings of fatigue or any other discomfort.

2. Attendant Risks and Discomforts
There exists the possibility of certain changes occurring during the test. They include abnormal blood pressure, fainting, irregular, fast or slow heart rhythm, and in rare instances, heart attack, stroke, or death. Every effort will be made to minimize these risks by evaluation of preliminary information relating to your health and fitness and by observations during testing. Emergency equipment and trained personnel are available to deal with unusual situations that may arise.

3. Responsibilities of the Participant
Information you possess about your health status or previous experiences of unusual feelings with physical effort may affect the safety and value of your exercise test. Your prompt reporting of feelings with effort during the exercise test itself is also of great importance. You are responsible for fully disclosing such information when requested by the testing staff.

4. Benefits to be Expected
The results obtained from the exercise test may assist in the diagnosis of your illness or in evaluating what type of physical activities you might do with low risk.

Continued on Next Page

Informed Consent *Continued*

5. Inquiries
Any questions about the procedures used in the exercise test or the results of your test are encouraged. If you have any concerns or questions, please ask us for further explanations.

6. Freedom of Consent
Your permission to perform this exercise test is voluntary. You are free to stop the test at any point, if you so desire.

I have read this form, and I understand the test procedures that I will perform and the attendant risks and discomforts. Knowing these risks and discomforts, and having had an opportunity to ask questions that have been answered to my satisfaction, I consent to participate in this test.

Date	
	Signature of Patient

Date	
	Signature of Witness

Date	
	Signature of physician or authorized delegate

Informed Consent for an Outpatient Cardiac Rehabilitation Program (Sample)

1. Explanation of Outpatient Cardiac Rehabilitation Program
You will be placed in a rehabilitation program that will include physical exercises, educational activities, and other health-related services. The levels of exercise which you will undertake will be based on your cardiovascular response to an exercise test. You will be given clear instructions regarding the amount and kind of regular exercise you should do. Your exercise sessions may be adjusted by the program staff and physician, depending on your progress. You will be given the opportunity for re-evaluation with a graded exercise test _____ months after the initiation of the rehabilitation program, and _____ months thereafter. Other retests may be recommended as needed.

Continued on Next Page

Informed Consent *Continued*

2. Monitoring
Your blood pressure will be monitored as required. You agree to learn how to count your own pulse rate and record it before, during, and after each exercise session, as instructed by program staff members.

3. Attendant Risks and Discomforts
There exists the possibility of certain changes occurring during exercise sessions. These include abnormal blood pressure, fainting, irregular, fast, or slow heart rhythm, and in rare instances, heart attack, stroke, or death. Every effort will be made to minimize those risks by provision of appropriate supervision during exercise. Emergency equipment and trained personnel are available to deal with unusual situations that may arise.

4. Benefits to be Expected
Participation in the rehabilitation program may help to evaluate which activities you may safely engage in during your daily life. No assurance can be given that the rehabilitation program will increase your functional capacity, although widespread evidence indicates improvement is usually achieved.

5. Responsibility of the Participant
To promote your safety and gain benefit, you must give priority to regular attendance and adherence to the prescribed intensity, duration, frequency, progression and type of activity. To achieve the best possible care:

A. DO <u>NOT</u>
• Withhold any information pertinent to symptoms from any staff member.
• Exceed your target heart rate.
• Exercise when you do not feel well.
• Exercise within 2 hours after eating or using tobacco products or alcohol.
• Use extremely hot water during showering after exercise (stay out of sauna, steam bath, and similar extreme temperatures).

B. DO
• Report any unusual symptoms that you experience before, during, or after exercise. (You may help assure the safety

Continued on Next Page

Informed Consent *Continued*

and well-being of others in the program if you would also report any unusual symptoms you notice in others.)

- Check in with the staff after showering/dressing before leaving the site.
- Follow, without exception, all recommendations made by staff concerning the limits on any exercise, weight control, or health-related activities which you may be encouraged to do and document by recordings.

6. Use of Medical Records

The information that is obtained during exercise testing and while you are a participant in the Cardiac Rehabilitation Program will be treated as privileged and confidential. It is not to be released or revealed to any person except your referring physician without your written consent. The information obtained, however, may be used for statistical analysis or scientific purposes with your right to privacy retained.

7. Inquiries

Any questions about the rehabilitation program are welcome. If you have any doubts or questions, please ask us for further explanation.

8. Freedom of Consent

Your permission to engage in the Cardiac Rehabilitation Program is voluntary. You are free to deny any consent if you so desire, both now and at any point in the program.

I acknowledge that I have read this form in its entirety or it has been read to me, and I understand the Rehabilitation Program in which I will be engaged. I accept the risks, rules, and regulations set forth. I understand the test procedures that I will perform and the attendant risks and discomforts. Knowing these, and having had an opportunity to ask questions which have been answered to my satisfaction, I consent to participate in this Rehabilitation Program.

_____

Signature of Patient

_____   _____

Date   Signature of Witness

Signature of physician or authorized delegate _____

prescription, that is, for experimental purposes, this should be indicated on the Informed Consent Form and applicable policies for the testing of human subjects must be implemented. A copy of the Policy on Human Subjects for Research is available from ACSM upon request.

Since most consent forms include a statement that emergency equipment is available, the program must ensure that available personnel are legally authorized to carry out emergency procedures which utilize such equipment. This is of particular importance when defibrillators are present, since use of defibrillators is limited to medical practitioners or others specifically authorized by law.

PATIENT INSTRUCTIONS

Explicit instructions for patients prior to exercise testing increase test validity and data accuracy. Whenever possible, written instructions along with a description of the evaluation should be provided well in advance of the appointment, so the patient can prepare adequately. The following points should be considered for inclusion in such preliminary instructions; however, specific instructions will vary with test type and purpose:

- Patients should refrain from ingesting food, alcohol, or caffeine or using tobacco products within 3 hours of testing.
- Patients should be rested for the assessment, avoiding significant exertion or exercise on the day of the assessment.
- Clothing should permit freedom of movement and include walking or running shoes. Women should bring a loose-fitting blouse with short sleeves that buttons down the front, and should avoid restrictive undergarments.

Continued on Next Page

- If the evaluation is on an outpatient basis, patients should be made aware that the evaluation may be fatiguing, and that they may wish to have someone accompany them to the assessment to drive home afterward.
- If the test is for diagnostic purposes, it may be helpful for patients to discontinue prescribed cardiovascular medications *only with physician* approval. Currently prescribed antianginal agents alter the hemodynamic response to exercise and significantly reduce the sensitivity of ECG changes for ischemia. Patients taking intermediate- or high-dose ß-blocking agents should taper their medication over a 2- to 4-day period to minimize hyperadrenergic withdrawal responses.
- If the test is for functional purposes, patients should continue their medication regimen on their usual schedule, so that the exercise responses will be consistent with responses expected during exercise training.
- Patients should bring a list of their medications to the assessment, including dosage and frequency of administration, and should report the last actual dose taken. As an alternative, patients may wish to bring their medications with them for the clinician to record.

REFERENCES

1. Fifth Report of the Joint Committee on Detection, Evaluation, and Treatment of High Blood Pressure (JNCV), *Arch. Int. Med.* 153:154–183, 1993.
2. Expert Panel on Detection, Evaluation, and Treatment of High Blood Cholesterol in Adults. Summary of the Second Report of the National Cholesterol Education Program (NCEP) Expert Panel on Detection, Evaluation, and Treatment of High Blood Cholesterol in Adults (Adult Treatment Panel II). *J Am Med Assoc* 269:3015–3023, 1993.
3. Miller A: *Pulmonary Function Tests in Clinical and Occupational Lung Disease.* Orlando: Grune & Stratton, 1986.
4. Wasserman K, Hansen JE, Sue DY and Whipp BJ: *Principles of Exercise Testing.* Philadelphia: Lea & Febiger, 1987, p. 79.
5. Hillegas EA and Sadowsky HS: Pulmonary diagnostic tests and procedures. In *Essentials of Cardiopulmonary Physical Therapy.* Philadelphia: WB Saunders, 1994.

chapter 4

PHYSICAL FITNESS TESTING

The term "physical fitness" has been defined in many ways. Most definitions of physical fitness refer strictly to the capacity for movement, and the following recently proposed definition is typical in this regard: *A set of attributes that people have or achieve that relates to the ability to perform physical activity.*[1] Such definitions are, by nature, rather broad and can be interpreted as encompassing an array of fitness components, some of which relate to athletic performance, but not health. Accordingly, the term "health-related physical fitness" has been used to denote fitness as it pertains to disease prevention and health promotion. One definition of health-related physical fitness is: *A state characterized by (a) an ability to perform daily activities with vigor, and (b) a demonstration of traits and capacities that are associated with low risk of premature development of the hypokinetic diseases (i.e., those associated with physical inactivity).*[2]

Although many different literal definitions of physical fitness have developed, there is relative uniformity in the *operational* definition of physical fitness. It has almost always been viewed as a multifactorial construct that includes several components. Each component is a movement-related trait or capacity that is considered to be largely independent of the others. *Health-related physical fitness* is typically defined as including cardiorespiratory endurance, body composition, muscular strength and endurance, and flexibility. The concept that underlies health-related physical fitness is that better status in each of the constituent components is associated with lower risk for development of disease and/or functional disability.

Note that informed consent procedures similar to those described in Chapter 3 must accompany fitness tests or groups of tests.

PURPOSES OF FITNESS TESTING

Measurement of physical fitness is a common and appropriate practice in preventive and rehabilitative exercise programs. The purposes of fitness testing in such programs include:

- Providing data that are helpful in development of exercise prescriptions
- Collecting baseline and follow-up data that allow evaluation of progress by exercise program participants
- Motivating participants by establishing reasonable and attainable fitness goals
- Educating participants about the concepts of physical fitness and individual fitness status
- Risk stratification

A fundamental goal of preventive and rehabilitative exercise programs is promotion of health. Therefore, such programs should focus on enhancement of the health-related components of physical fitness. This chapter provides guidelines for the measurement and evaluation of health-related physical fitness in presumably healthy adults.

BASIC PRINCIPLES AND GUIDELINES

The information obtained from physical fitness testing, in combination with the individual's health and medical information, can be used by the health/fitness professional to meet an individual's specific fitness needs. A sound, well-conducted physical fitness test measures what it purports to measure (i.e., is valid), is reliable, and is relatively inexpensive and easy to administer. Additionally, the test should yield results which can be directly and appropriately compared to normative data.

PRETEST INSTRUCTIONS

Before administering a physical fitness test, certain measures should be taken to ensure client safety. A minimal recommendation is that individuals complete a questionnaire such as the PAR-Q (see Chapter 2) prior to coming to the testing facility. Individuals should also be given precise instructions before they come to the testing facility. In general, individuals should be instructed to:

- Wear comfortable, loose-fitting clothing
- Drink plenty of fluids over the 24-hour period preceding the test
- Avoid food, tobacco, alcohol, and caffeine for 3 hours prior to taking the test
- Avoid exercise or strenuous physical activity the day of the test
- Get an adequate amount of sleep (6 to 8 hours) the night before the test

TEST ORDER

When multiple tests are to be administered, the organization of the testing session can be very important, depending on what physical fitness components are to be evaluated. If all components are assessed during a single session, body composition measures should be taken first, followed (in order) by tests of cardiorespiratory endurance, muscular fitness, and flexibility. Testing cardiorespiratory endurance after assessing muscular fitness (which elevates heart rate) can produce inaccurate results regarding an individual's cardiorespiratory endurance status—particularly when submaximal tests are used. Likewise, dehydration effects resulting from endurance tests may influence body composition measurements. If the testing protocol involves assessing resting measures (e.g., heart rate, blood pressure, and blood analysis), such measures should be taken before fitness testing begins.

TEST ENVIRONMENT

The test environment is important for test validity and reliability. Test anxiety, emotional problems, food in the stomach, bladder distention, climate variation, and pain should be controlled as much as possible. To minimize anxiety, the test environment should be quiet and private and the temperature of the room maintained at 70 to 74°F (21 to 23°C). The room should be equipped with a comfortable seat and/or examination table to be used for resting blood pressure and ECG recordings, in addition to the standard testing equipment required. The demeanor of personnel should be one of relaxed confidence so as to immediately put the subject at ease. Testing procedures should not be rushed, and all procedures must be clearly explained prior to initiating the process. These seemingly minor tasks are easily accomplished and will assist in achieving valid test results.

BODY COMPOSITION

Evaluation of body composition is a common and important component of overall physical fitness assessment. It is well-established that excess body fat is harmful to health, but many misconceptions exist regarding the assessment and interpretation of such data. Surveys by the U.S. National Center for Health Statistics show that nearly 50% of adult women in the U.S. report that they are dieting to lose weight[3]; however, only about 25% of women are at increased health risk from being overweight according to standards established by the U.S. Surgeon General.

Body composition refers to the relative percentages of body weight comprised of fat and fat-free body tissue. Body composition can be estimated using both laboratory and field techniques. Different assessment techniques are briefly reviewed in this section. Specific instructions for obtaining measurements and calculating estimates of body fat are beyond the scope of this text, but a more detailed description is provided in the *Resource Manual for Guidelines for Exercise Testing and Prescription, 2nd edition*.

With all body composition measurement techniques, the technician must be well-trained, routinely practice the techniques, and demonstrate reliability in his/her measurements before collecting actual data.

HYDROSTATIC WEIGHING

Hydrostatic (underwater) weighing[4,5] is commonly considered to be the criterion measurement technique for assessing body composition. This technique is based on Archimedes' principle, which states that when a body is immersed in water, it will be buoyed by a counterforce equal to the weight of the water displaced. Bone and muscle tissue are more dense than water, whereas fat tissue is less dense. Therefore, a person with more fat-free body mass for the same total body weight weighs more in water, has a higher body density, and lower percentage of body fat. While hydrostatic weighing is the standard, there are several sources of error inherent in the procedure. First, a measure or estimation of lung residual volume is needed to calculate body density. Second, the great variability in bone density among individuals is not accounted for by this method. Finally, hydrostatic weighing requires expensive, special equipment, and the procedure is somewhat complicated and time-consuming. For some individuals, submersion of the head underwater may be difficult or anxiety-provoking.

Body density can be derived from the following formula:

$$\text{Body Density} = \frac{\text{Weight in air}}{\left[\dfrac{(\text{Weight in air} - \text{Weight in water})}{\text{Density of water}} - \dfrac{\text{Residual}}{\text{Volume}}\right]}$$

Prediction equations are then used to convert body density into percent body fat. The two most commonly used formulas that yield similar body fat values are:[6, 7]

$$\% \text{ fat} = (457/\text{Body Density}) - 414.2^*$$

$$\% \text{ fat} = (495/\text{Body Density}) - 450^\dagger$$

*Equation from Reference 6.
†Equation from Reference 7.

SKINFOLD MEASUREMENTS

Body composition determined from skinfold measurements correlates well ($r \geq 0.80$) with body composition determined by hydrostatic weighing. The principle behind this technique is that the amount of subcutaneous fat is proportional to (about 50% of) the total amount of body fat. Table 4–1 presents a standardized description of skinfold sites and procedures.

Various regression equations have been developed to predict body density from skinfold measurements. However, many of the regression equations used are specific to the populations from which they were derived. A relatively recent trend has been to develop generalized rather than population-specific equations. These equations have been developed using regression models that take into consideration data from several different research studies, the main advantage being that one generalized equation can be substituted for several population-specific equations without a loss in prediction accuracy for a wide range of individuals. Table 4–2 contains some of the more commonly used generalized skinfold equations.[8]

ANTHROPOMETRIC METHODS

Anthropometry includes measures such as height, weight, and circumferences (girths) of various body segments or areas. These simple measurements provide a practical and inexpensive alternative for estimating body composition and are commonly used in clinical and fitness settings. Results are not as accurate, however, as those derived from hydrostatic weighing.

Several prediction equations have been developed utilizing circumference measurements in combination with skinfold measures. Various limb and body girths are mea-

TABLE 4–1. STANDARDIZED DESCRIPTION OF SKINFOLD SITES AND PROCEDURES

Skinfold Site	Description
Abdominal	Vertical fold; 2 cm to the right side of the umbilicus
Triceps	Vertical fold; on the posterior midline of the upper arm, halfway between the acromion and olecranon processes, with the arm held freely to the side of the body
Biceps	Vertical fold; on the anterior aspect of the arm over the belly of the biceps muscle, 1 cm above the level used to mark the triceps site
Chest/Pectoral	Diagonal fold; one-half the distance between the anterior axillary line and the nipple (men) or one-third of the distance between the anterior axillary line and the nipple (women)
Medial Calf	Vertical fold; at the maximum circumference of the calf on the midline of its medial border
Midaxillary	Vertical fold; on the midaxillary line at the level of the xiphoid process of the sternum. (An alternate method is a horizontal fold taken at the level of the xiphoid/sternal border in the midaxillary line.)
Subscapular	Diagonal fold (at a 45° angle); 1 to 2 cm below the inferior angle of the scapula
Suprailiac	Diagonal fold; in line with the natural angle of the iliac crest taken in the anterior axillary line immediately superior to the iliac crest
Thigh	Vertical fold; on the anterior midline of the thigh, midway between the proximal border of the patella and the inguinal crease (hip)

Procedures

- All measurements should be made on the right side of the body
- Caliper should be placed 1 cm away from the thumb and finger, perpendicular to the skinfold, and halfway between the crest and the base of the fold
- Pinch should be maintained while reading the caliper
- Wait 1 to 2 seconds (and not longer) before reading caliper
- Take duplicate measures at each site and retest if duplicate measurements are not within 1 to 2 mm
- Rotate through measurement sites or allow time for skin to regain normal texture and thickness

TABLE 4–2. GENERALIZED SKINFOLD EQUATIONS*

Men

7-Site Formula (chest, midaxillary, triceps, subscapular, abdomen, suprailiac, thigh)

Body Density = 1.112 − 0.00043499 *(Sum of Seven Skinfolds)* + 0.00000055 *(Sum of Seven Skinfolds)*^{2} − 0.00028826 *(Age)*

4-Site Formula (abdomen, suprailiac, triceps, thigh)

Percent Body Fat = 0.29288 *(Sum of Four Skinfolds)* − 0.0005 *(Sum of Four Skinfolds)*^{2} + 0.15845 *(Age)* − 5.76377

3-Site Formulas

Body Density = 1.1093800 − 0.0008267 *(Sum of Three Skinfolds)* + 0.0000016 *(Sum of Three Skinfolds)*^{2} − 0.000257 *(Age)* (chest, abdomen, thigh)
Body Density = 1.1125025 − 0.0013125 *(Sum of Three Skinfolds)* + 0.0000055 *(Sum of Three Skinfolds)*^{2} − 0.0002440 *(Age)* (chest, triceps, subscapular)
Percent Body Fat = 0.39287 *(Sum of Three Skinfolds)* − 0.00105 *(Sum of Three Skinfolds)*^{2} + 0.15772 *(Age)* − 5.18845 (abdomen, suprailiac, triceps)

Women

7-Site Formula (chest, midaxillary, triceps, subscapular, abdomen, suprailiac, thigh)

Body Density = 1.0970 − 0.00046971 *(Sum of Seven Skinfolds)* + 0.00000056 *(Sum of Seven Skinfolds)*^{2} − 0.00012828 *(Age)*

4-Site Formula (abdomen, suprailiac, triceps, thigh)

Percent Body Fat − 0.29669 *(Sum of Four Skinfolds)* − 0.00043 *(Sum of Four Skinfolds)*^{2} + 0.02963 *(Age)* + 1.4072

3-Site Formulas

Percent Body Fat = 0.41563 *(Sum of Three Skinfolds*; triceps, abdomen, suprailiac) − 0.00112 *(Sum of Three Skinfolds)*^{2} + 0.03661 *(Age)* + 4.03653
Body Density = 1.0994921 − 0.0009929 *(Sum of Three Skinfolds;* triceps, suprailiac, thigh) + 0.0000023 *(Sum of Three Skinfolds)*^{2} − 0.0001392 *(Age)*

Note: The researchers who developed these equations used vertical instead of horizontal skinfolds at the abdominal and midaxillary sites.
*Adapted from Reference 8.

sured (Table 4–3) and used in equations that predict body density or fat-free body mass.

The Body Mass Index (BMI), or Quetelet Index, is used to assess weight relative to height and is calculated by dividing body weight in kilograms by height in meters

TABLE 4–3. STANDARDIZED DESCRIPTION OF CIRCUMFERENCE SITES AND PROCEDURES

Circumference Site	Description
Abdomen	At the level of the umbilicus
Calf	At the maximum circumference between the knee and the ankle
Forearm	With the arms hanging downward but slightly away from the trunk and palms facing forward, at the maximal forearm circumference
Hips	At the maximal circumference of the hips or buttocks region, whichever is larger (above the gluteal fold)
Arm	With the subject's arm to the side of the body, midway between the acromion and olecranon processes
Waist	At the narrowest part of the torso (above the umbilicus and below the xiphoid process)
Thigh	With the subject's legs slightly apart, at the maximal circumference of the thigh (below the gluteal fold)

Procedures

- All limb measurements should be taken on the right side of the body using a tension-regulated tape
- The subject should stand erect but relaxed
- Place the tape perpendicular to the long axis of the body part in each case
- Pull the tape to proper tension without pinching skin
- Take duplicate measures at each site and retest if duplicate measurements are not within 7 mm or 0.25 in

squared (wt/ht^2). An individual's BMI can be easily determined through the use of a nomogram[9] (Fig. 4–1). BMI is a relatively good indicator of total body composition in population-based studies and is related to health outcomes. A major limitation of BMI is that it is difficult to interpret to clients, and to project changes in actual weight loss to BMI changes. The Panel on Energy, Obesity, and Body Weight Standards has recommended that the following table be used when classifying obesity according to BMI values:[10]

20–24.9 kg/m^2	Desirable range for adult men and women
25–29.9 kg/m^2	Grade 1 obesity
30–40 kg/m^2	Grade 2 obesity
>40 kg/m^2	Grade 3 obesity (morbid obesity)

Obesity-related health risks begin in the BMI range of 25 to 30 kg/m^2.

Recent data indicate that the pattern of body fat distribution is an important predictor of the health risks of obesity.[11] Individuals with more fat on the trunk, especially abdominal fat, are at increased risk of hypertension, Type II diabetes, hyperlipidemia, CAD, and premature death when compared to individuals who are equally fat, but have more of their fat on the extremities. The waist-to-hip ratio (WHR—the circumference of the waist divided by the circumference of the hips) is a simple method for determining body fat pattern.[12] Ratios above 0.95 for men and 0.86 for women place the individual at significantly increased health risk of disease. A nomogram for determining the WHR is provided in Figure 4–2.[11]

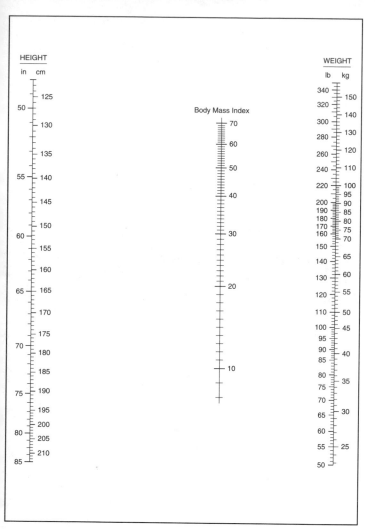

FIG. 4–1. The Body Mass Index (kg/m²) is calculated from this nomogram by reading the central scale after a straightedge is placed between height and body weight. Reprinted with permission from Reference 9.

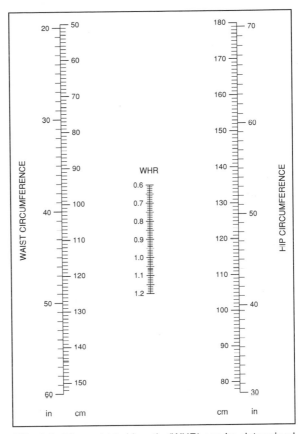

FIG. 4–2. The waist-to-hip ratio (WHR) can be determined by placing a straightedge between the column for waist circumference and the column for hip circumference and reading the ratio from the point where this straightedge crosses the WHR line. The waist circumference is the smallest circumference below the rib cage and above the navel, and the hip circumference is taken as the largest circumference at the posterior extension of the buttocks. Reprinted with permission from Reference 12.

BIA AND INFRARED INTERACTANCE

Many other methods are currently being used to assess body composition. Additional research is needed, however, to establish their reliability and validity. Two techniques which appear to have promise are bioelectrical impedance analysis (BIA) and infrared interactance.

BIA involves passing a small electric current through the body and measuring the resistance encountered. Fat-free tissue is a good conductor of electrical current, whereas fat is not. The resistance to current flow is thus inversely related to fat-free mass. In general, body composition results from BIA are less accurate and require more assumptions than those obtained through accurate skinfold measurements. To reduce measurement errors associated with BIA, the following procedural guidelines are recommended:

- Abstain from eating or drinking within 4 hours of the assessment
- Avoid moderate or vigorous physical activity within 12 hours of the assessment
- Void completely before the assessment
- Abstain from alcohol consumption within 48 hours of the assessment
- Ingest no diuretic agents prior to the assessment unless prescribed by a physician

A major limitation of BIA is the fact that it consistently overestimates percent body fat in very lean individuals and underestimates percent body fat in obese individuals.[8,13] Despite this limitation, however, BIA holds promise as a very convenient, easy to administer, noninvasive and safe method of assessing body composition in a fitness setting.

Infrared interactance is based on the principles of light absorption and reflection using near-infrared spectroscopy to provide information about the chemical composition of the body. Further research is needed to develop and cross-validate gender-specific equations for infrared interactance, and to determine whether this technique is an accurate method for assessing body composition.

CARDIORESPIRATORY ENDURANCE

Cardiorespiratory endurance is defined as the ability to perform large muscle, dynamic, moderate-to-high intensity exercise for prolonged periods. Performance of such exercise depends on the functional state of the respiratory, cardiovascular, and skeletal muscle systems. Cardiorespiratory endurance is considered health-related because (a) low levels of fitness have been associated with markedly increased risk of premature death from all causes and specifically from cardiovascular disease, and (b) higher fitness is associated with higher levels of habitual physical activity, which is, in turn, associated with many health benefits.

THE CONCEPT OF $\dot{V}O_{2max}$

The traditionally accepted criterion measure of cardiorespiratory endurance is directly measured maximal oxygen uptake ($\dot{V}O_{2max}$). Measurement of $\dot{V}O_{2max}$ involves analysis of expired air samples collected while the subject performs exercise of progressing intensity. Detailed descriptions of recommended procedures for direct measurement of $\dot{V}O_2$ and $\dot{V}O_{2max}$ are provided in Appendix D. For the purpose of evaluating cardiorespiratory endurance, $\dot{V}O_{2max}$ values are typically expressed relative to body weight (i.e., $ml \cdot kg^{-1} \cdot min^{-1}$) (see also Appendix D).

Because direct measurement of $\dot{V}O_{2max}$ is often not feasible, many procedures for estimation of $\dot{V}O_{2max}$ have been developed (see Appendix D). These tests have been validated by examining: (a) the correlation between directly measured $\dot{V}O_{2max}$ and the $\dot{V}O_{2max}$ estimated from physiologic responses to submaximal exercise (e.g., heart rate at a specified power output), or (b) the correlation between directly measured $\dot{V}O_{2max}$ and test performance (e.g., time to run 1 mile or time to volitional fatigue using a standard test protocol).

MAXIMAL VS. SUBMAXIMAL EXERCISE TESTING

While maximal-effort tests must be used to measure $\dot{V}O_{2max}$, submaximal exercise tests can be used to estimate $\dot{V}O_{2max}$. The decision to select a maximal or submaximal exercise test largely depends upon the reasons for the test, the type of subject to be tested, and the availability of appropriate equipment and personnel. $\dot{V}O_{2max}$ can be measured during maximal exercise testing by direct analysis of expired gases or estimated from maximal exercise intensity using prediction equations (Appendix D). Direct analysis of expired gases yields the most accurate determination of $\dot{V}O_{2max}$. This method, however, is costly (in terms of equipment), requires specially trained personnel and tends to be time-consuming. For these reasons, direct measurement of $\dot{V}O_{2max}$ is generally reserved for research or clinical settings. Estimating $\dot{V}O_{2max}$ from maximal exercise intensity is considered to be the next most accurate method. It has the disadvantage, however, of requiring participants to exercise to the point of volitional fatigue. Compared to submaximal exercise tests, maximal exercise tests are more useful clinically in aiding in the diagnosis of CAD in asymptomatic individuals.

Since maximal exercise testing is not a feasible method of assessing cardiorespiratory endurance for the vast majority of health/fitness practitioners, submaximal exercise tests were developed. The basic aim of submaximal exercise testing is to determine the relationship between a subject's heart rate response and his/her $\dot{V}O_2$ during progressive exercise and use that relationship to predict $\dot{V}O_{2max}$. In order to accurately determine this relationship, heart rate and $\dot{V}O_2$ need to be measured at two or more submaximal exercise intensities. Alternately, HR can be plotted against exercise intensity as in Figure 4–3, and $\dot{V}O_2$ estimated from the intensity as in Appendix D.

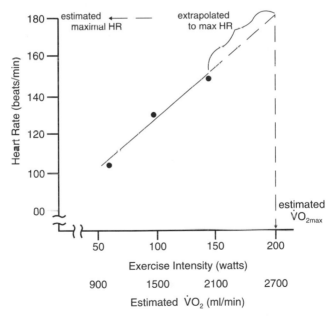

FIG. 4–3. Heart rate obtained from at least two (more are preferable) submaximal exercise intensities may be extrapolated to the age-predicted maximal heart rate. A vertical line to the intensity scale estimates maximal exercise intensity from which an estimated $\dot{V}O_{2max}$ can be calculated (see Appendix D).

Submaximal exercise tests make several assumptions:

- That a steady-state heart rate is obtained for each exercise work rate
- That a linear relationship exists between heart rate and oxygen uptake (or work rate if VO_2 is not measured)
- That the maximal heart rate for a given age is uniform
- That mechanical efficiency (i.e., VO_2 at a given work rate) is the same for everyone

These assumptions are usually not fully met, however, and this contributes to errors in predicting $\dot{V}O_{2max}$. Submaximal exercise testing, though not as precise as maximal exercise testing, can still provide a reasonably accurate reflection of an individual's fitness without the cost, risk, time, and effort on the part of the subject. If an individual is given repeated submaximal exercise tests over a period of weeks or months and the heart rate response to a fixed work rate decreases over time, it is likely that the individual's cardiorespiratory fitness has improved, irrespective of the accuracy of the $\dot{V}O_{2max}$ prediction.

DISCONTINUOUS (INTERMITTENT) VS. CONTINUOUS PROTOCOLS

Continuous and discontinuous protocols are available for both maximal and submaximal testing on a variety of testing modalities. Continuous protocols consist of progressive stages of increasing work intensities with no rest intervals. Discontinuous protocols alternate work and rest intervals. As a result, a plateau in $\dot{V}O_2$ with increasing exercise intensity (i.e., $\dot{V}O_{2max}$) occurs more often, in part because the subject does not experience the degree of local muscular fatigue as with continuous protocols. Although intermittent protocols are advantageous for some populations or conditions, they take much longer to administer. This time requirement is a major limitation in most settings resulting in the use of continuous protocols for routine exercise testing.

USE OF SUBJECTIVE RATING SCALES

Rating of perceived exertion (RPE) has been found to be a valuable and reliable indicator in monitoring an individual's exercise tolerance. Often used while conducting graded exercise tests, perceived exertion ratings correlate highly with measured exercise heart rates and calculated oxygen consumption values. Borg's[14] RPE scale was developed to allow the exerciser to subjectively rate his/ her feelings during exercise, taking into account personal fitness level, environmental conditions, and general fatigue levels. Currently, two RPE scales are widely used: the original, which rates exercise intensity on a scale of 6 to 20, and the revised scale of 0 to 10. This revised and simplified scale uses terminology better understood by the subject, thereby providing the tester with more valid information by which to further direct the test. Both scales account for the linear increase in Vo_2 and heart rate during exercise, while the revised scale also considers the nonlinear responses of variables such as blood lactic acid accumulation and ventilation.

The greatest value of the RPE scale is that it provides exercisers of all fitness levels with easily understood guidelines regarding exercise intensity. It has been found that a cardiorespiratory training effect and the threshold for blood lactate accumulation are achieved at a rating of "somewhat hard" or "hard," which corresponds to a rating of 13 to 16 on the original scale or 4 to 5 on the

TABLE 4–4. ORIGINAL AND REVISED SCALES FOR RATINGS OF PERCEIVED EXERTION (RPE)*

Original Scale		Revised Scale	
6		0	Nothing at all
7	Very, very light	0.5	Very, very weak
8		1	Very weak
9	Very light	2	Weak
10		3	Moderate
11	Fairly light	4	Somewhat strong
12		5	Strong
13	Somewhat hard	6	
14		7	Very strong
15	Hard	8	
16		9	
17	Very hard	10	Very, very strong
18		•	Maximal
19	Very, very hard		
20			

*From Reference 14.

revised scale. The original and revised RPE scales are shown in Table 4–4.

MODE OF TESTING

Submaximal cycle ergometer tests. Submaximal cycle ergometer tests are popular assessment techniques for cardiorespiratory endurance. The YMCA protocol uses two to four, 3-minute stages of continuous exercise (see Figure 4–4). The test is designed to raise the steady state heart rate of the subject to 110 to 150 beats/min for two consecutive stages. An important point to remember is that two consecutive heart rate measurements must be obtained in the 110 to 150 beats/min range to predict $\dot{V}O_{2max}$. In the YMCA protocol, each work rate is performed for 3 minutes, with heart rates recorded during the final 15 to 30 seconds of the second and third minutes. If these heart

YMCA Cycle Ergometry Protocol

1st Stage	150 kgm/min (0.5 kg)

	HR < 80	HR 80–89	HR 90–100	HR > 100
2nd Stage	750 kgm/min (2.5 kg)*	600 kgm/min (2.0 kg)	450 kgm/min (1.5 kg)	300 kgm/min (1.0 kg)
3rd Stage	900 kgm/min (3.0 kg)	750 kgm/min (2.5 kg)	600 kgm/min (2.0 kg)	450 kgm/min (1.5 kg)
4th Stage	1050 kgm/min (3.5 kg)	900 kgm/min (3.0 kg)	750 kgm/min (2.5 kg)	600 kgm/min (2.0 kg)

Directions

1. Set the first work rate at 150 kgm/min (0.5 kg at 50 rpm)
2. If the HR in the third minute of the stage is:

    less than (<) 80, set the second stage at 750 kgm/min (2.5 kg at 50 rpm)
    80-90, set the second stage at 600 kgm/min (2.0 kg at 50 rpm)
    90-100, set the second stage at 450 kgm/min (1.5 kg at 50 rpm)
    greater than (>) 100, set the second stage at 300 kgm/min (1.0 kg at 50 rpm)

3. Set the third and fourth (if required) stages according to the work rates in the columns below the second loads.

FIG. 4–4. YMCA cycle ergometry protocol; *resistance settings shown here are appropriate for an ergometer with a 6 m/rev flywheel.

TABLE 4–5. GENERAL PROCEDURES FOR SUBMAXIMAL TESTING OF CARDIORESPIRATORY ENDURANCE USING A CYCLE ERGOMETER

1. The exercise test should begin with a 2- to 3-minute warm-up in order to acquaint the client with the cycle ergometer and prepare him/her for the exercise intensity in the first stage of the test
2. The specific protocol consists of 3-minute stages with appropriate increments in work rate
3. The client should be properly positioned on the cycle ergometer (i.e., upright posture, 5° bend in the knee at maximal leg extension, hands in proper position on handlebars)
4. Heart rate should be monitored at least two times during each stage, near the end of the second and third minutes of each stage. If HR > 110 beats/min, steady state heart rate (i.e., 2 HRs within ±6 beats/min) should be reached before the work rate is increased
5. Blood pressure should be monitored in the later portion of each stage
6. RPE should be monitored near the end of each stage using either the 6–20 or the 0–10 scale
7. Client appearance and symptoms should be monitored regularly
8. The test should be terminated when the subject reaches 85% of age-predicted maximal HR (70% of HR reserve), fails to conform to the exercise test protocol, experiences signs of excessive discomfort, or an emergency situation arises
9. An appropriate cool-down/recovery period should be initiated consisting of either:
   a. continued pedaling at a work rate equivalent to that of the first stage of the exercise test protocol or lower; or,
   b. a passive cool-down if the subject experiences signs of discomfort or an emergency situation occurs
10. All observations (HR, BP, RPE, client signs and symptoms) should be continued for at least 4 minutes of recovery unless abnormal responses occur which would warrant a longer post-test observation

rates are not within 5 beats/min of each other, then that work rate is maintained for an additional minute. Standardized procedures used in the ACSM Health/Fitness Instructor$_{SM}$ examination are presented in Table 4–5. The heart rate measured during the last minute of each stage is plotted against work rate. The line generated from the plotted points is then extended to the age-predicted maximal heart rate. A corresponding maximal work rate and $\dot{V}O_{2max}$ can then be estimated.

The Åstrand-Ryhming cycle ergometer test is a single-stage test lasting 6 minutes.[15] The suggested work rate is selected based upon gender and an individual's activity status as follows: males—unconditioned, 300 or 600 kgm/min (50 or 100 watts), or conditioned, 600 or 900 kgm/min (100 or 150 watts); females—unconditioned, 300 or 450 kgm/min (50 or 75 watts), or conditioned, 450 or 600 kgm/min (75 or 100 watts). The pedal rate is set at 50 rpm. Heart rate is measured during the 5th and 6th minutes of work. The average of the two heart rates is then used to estimate $\dot{V}O_{2max}$ from a nomogram (Figure 4–5). This value must then be corrected for age differences using the following correction factors:[16]

Age	Correction Factor
15	1.10
25	1.00
35	0.87
40	0.83
45	0.78
50	0.75
55	0.71
60	0.68
65	0.65

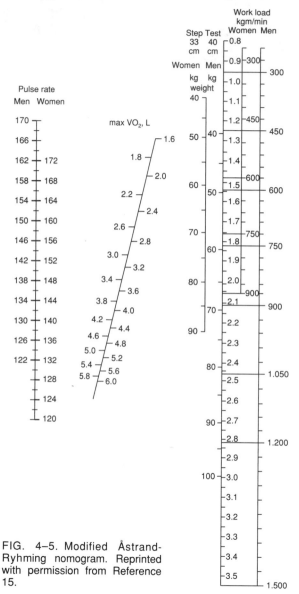

FIG. 4–5. Modified Åstrand-Ryhming nomogram. Reprinted with permission from Reference 15.

Submaximal treadmill tests. The primary exercise modality for submaximal exercise testing has traditionally been the cycle ergometer, although in many settings, treadmills have been used. Submaximal treadmill testing often uses an endpoint based on a predetermined heart rate (HR), usually 85% of predicted maximal heart rate reserve (i.e., [(maximal HR − resting HR) (0.85)] + resting HR). The most frequently employed protocols for submaximal treadmill testing are the Bruce and Balke protocols (Figure 4–6). It is recommended that an electrocardiograph, heart rate monitor, or a stethoscope be used to determine heart rate.

Step tests. The 3-Minute Step Test is a test that has been used for mass testing. According to the YMCA protocol,[17,18] the test is to be conducted on a 12-inch high bench, with a stepping rate of 24 steps/min for 3 minutes. After exercise is completed, the subject immediately sits down and heart rate is counted for 1 minute. Counting must start within 5 seconds of the end of exercise. Using this heart rate, a qualitative rating of fitness can be determined using published normative tables.[18]

Field tests Two of the most widely used running tests for assessing cardiorespiratory endurance are the Cooper 12-minute test and the 1.5 mile test for time. The objective in the 12-minute test is to cover the greatest distance in the allotted time period. The objective for the 1.5-mile test is to run the distance in as short a period of time as possible. Normative data are available to provide a reasonably accurate estimate of $\dot{V}O_{2max}$ of the individual who has been tested (see Appendix D).

One of the most positive features of these tests is that they are very easy to administer. On the other hand, such performance-based tests have a few substantial limitations. For example, an individual's level of motivation and pacing ability can have a profound impact on that person's test results. Of greater potential importance, a

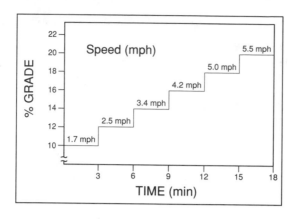

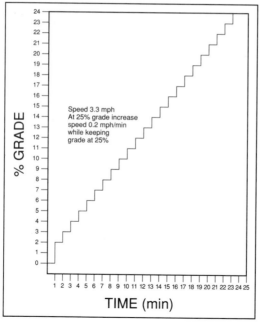

FIG. 4–6. The Bruce (upper panel) and Balke (lower panel) tread-mill graded exercise test protocols.

certain degree of risk exists during such testing since individuals are encouraged to put forth a maximal effort.

In recent years, the Rockport One-Mile Fitness Walking Test has gained wide popularity as an effective means for estimating cardiorespiratory endurance. The primary task involved in this assessment procedure is to have an individual walk 1 mile as fast as possible, preferably on a track or a level surface. Immediately upon completion of walking, the individual's HR is measured using a 15-second pulse count. VO_{2max} is estimated from a regression equation based on weight, age, gender, walk time, and postexercise HR (see Table D–3, Appendix D).

TEST SEQUENCE AND MEASURES

After the initial screening process, selected baseline measurements should be obtained prior to the start of the exercise test. Whenever possible, participants should have a resting ECG evaluated before engaging in an exercise test, although this is not a requirement for apparently healthy individuals. At a minimum, resting (pre-exercise) HR and blood pressure (BP) should be obtained during the period immediately preceding the exercise test. HR, BP, and RPE should be obtained at regular intervals during the exercise test with continuous hemodynamic monitoring during the recovery period. HR and BP should be measured during each stage of the exercise testing protocol (typically every 2 or 3 minutes) and at 1- or 2- minute intervals during the recovery period. The recovery period should consist of 3 to 5 minutes of low-intensity exercise [e.g., walking at 2 to 3 mph, low-load (75 to 150 kgm/min) cycling, etc.]. This period of low-intensity exercise should last until HR and BP stabilize, but not necessarily until they reach pre-exercise levels.

HR can be determined using several techniques, including radial or carotid pulse palpation, auscultation with a stethoscope, or the use of pulse monitors. The pulse pal-pation technique involves "feeling" the pulse by placing the first and second fingers over an artery (usually the radial artery located near the thumbside of the wrist or the carotid artery located in the neck near the larynx). The heart beats are typically counted for either 10 or 15 seconds, and then multiplied by 6 or 4, respectively, to determine the per-minute HR. When palpating the carotid artery, heavy pressure should not be applied because pressure over baroreceptors in the carotid arteries may cause a reflex slowing of the heart rate. For the auscultation method, the bell of the stethoscope should be placed to the left of the sternum just above the level of the nipple. The auscultation method is most accurate when the heart sounds are clearly audible and the subject's torso is relatively stable. Over the years, several automated heart rate monitors have been developed. Heart rate monitors using chest electrodes have proven to be accurate and reliable, provided there is no outside electrical interference (e.g., emissions from the display consoles of computerized exercise equipment).

BP should be measured with the subject's arm relaxed and not grasping a handrail (treadmill or stair-climbing machine) or handlebar (cycle ergometer). To help ensure accurate readings, the use of an appropriate-sized blood pressure cuff is important. The rubber bladder of the blood pressure cuff should encircle at least two-thirds of the subject's upper arm. If the subject's arm is large, a normal-size adult cuff will be too small, making the readings higher than they actually are (the converse is also true). Blood pressure measurements should be taken with a mercury sphygmomanometer adjusted to eye level or a recently calibrated aneroid manometer. Standards for the measurement of blood pressure are published by the American Heart Association.

During exercise testing, rating of perceived exertion can be used as an indication of impending fatigue. Most subjects reach their subjective limit of fatigue at an RPE of 18 to 19 (very, very hard) or 9 to 10 (very, very strong) on the 0 to 10 scale; therefore, RPE can effectively be used to monitor progress toward maximal exertion during exercise testing. Clinical and practical experience indicate, however, that approximately 5 to 10% of individuals will tend to underestimate RPE during the early and middle stages of an exercise test. It is important to use standardized instructions to reduce problems of misinterpretation of RPE. The following are recommended instructions for using the RPE scale during exercise testing:

> "During the exercise test we want you to pay close attention to how hard you feel the exercise work rate is. This feeling should reflect your total amount of exertion and fatigue, combining all sensations and feelings of physical stress, effort, and fatigue. Don't concern yourself with any one factor such as leg pain, shortness of breath or exercise intensity, but try to concentrate on your total, inner feeling of exertion. Try not to underestimate or overestimate your feeling of exertion; be as accurate as you can."

TEST TERMINATION CRITERIA

Graded exercise testing, whether maximal or submaximal, is a safe procedure when subject screening and testing guidelines (see Chapter 2) are adhered to. Occasionally, for safety reasons the test should be terminated prior to the subject reaching a measured $\dot{V}O_{2max}$, volitional fatigue, or a predetermined endpoint. General indications—those which do not rely on physician involvement or ECG monitoring—for stopping an exercise test are outlined in Table 4–6. More specific termination criteria for clinical or diagnostic testing are provided in Chapter 5.

TABLE 4–6. GENERAL INDICATIONS FOR STOPPING AN EXERCISE TEST IN APPARENTLY HEALTHY ADULTS*

1. Onset of angina or angina-like symptoms
2. Significant drop (20 mm Hg) in systolic blood pressure or a failure of the systolic blood pressure to rise with an increase in exercise intensity
3. Excessive rise in blood pressure: systolic pressure >260 mm Hg or diastolic pressure >115 mm Hg
4. Signs of poor perfusion: lightheadedness, confusion, ataxia, pallor, cyanosis, nausea, or cold and clammy skin
5. Failure of heart rate to increase with increased exercise intensity
6. Noticeable change in heart rhythm
7. Subject requests to stop
8. Physical or verbal manifestations of severe fatigue
9. Failure of the testing equipment

*Assumes that testing is nondiagnostic and is being performed without direct physician involvement or electrocardiographic monitoring. For clinical testing, Table 5–4 provides more definitive and specific termination criteria.

MUSCULAR FITNESS

The term "muscular fitness" has been used to describe the integrated status of muscular strength and muscular endurance. If properly conducted, programs for the development of muscular fitness can help maintain or improve posture and prevent or reduce muscular low back pain. Maintenance of adequate levels of muscular fitness is also an important consideration with regard to the capacity of the elderly to perform essential daily tasks and to live independently.

Regardless of which component of muscular fitness (muscular strength or muscular endurance) is to be tested, a number of factors must be taken into consideration, including: [9]

- The devices commonly employed to assess muscular fitness all have design features and usage requirements that make the test results less than 100% reliable. For example, if the device has a pad that the subject pushes against, the extent to which the pad is depressed affects the measurement. Also, if procedures require that the body must be in an exact position, it may be difficult to achieve the same position each time a person is tested. Measuring muscular fitness is not a process that involves unequivocal precision. Knowing the design limitations of the device used, as well as the potential problems that might occur with any deviation in the protocol for using the device, enables one to be better prepared to interpret the results that are obtained.

- Muscular strength and muscular endurance are specific to the muscle or muscle group, the type of muscular contraction (static or dynamic—concentric, eccentric, isokinetic), the speed of muscular contraction (slow or fast), and the joint angle being tested (static contraction). Accordingly, the results of any one test are specific to the specific parameters of the procedure used to obtain the measurement. No single test exists for evaluating total body muscular strength or muscular endurance.

- The test items used to measure either muscular strength or muscular endurance should be selected with care. The most appropriate tests for measuring muscular endurance are those which are proportional to the body weight or the maximum strength level of the individual being tested.

- Because muscular fitness is often directly related to both the total body weight and the amount of lean muscle mass of the individual being tested, the test results should be expressed in relative terms (e.g., N/kg body weight or kg/kg body weight). The value of expressing muscular fitness test results in relative terms is particularly worthwhile when comparing one individual to another or one group to another.

- Because most muscular fitness tests require a maximal effort, care should be taken to control those factors that might affect maximal performance. Among the factors that could influence how well an individual performs are: time of day, fatigue, medication, motivation level, and emotional state. Steps should be taken to ensure that the maximal effort being exerted does not subject the individual to an unsafe level of exertion.

> • Caution should be used when comparing the results of the muscular fitness testing to normative data. Much of the normative data relating to muscular fitness is either outdated, invalid, or unreliable to varying degrees.

MUSCULAR STRENGTH

Muscular strength refers to the maximal force (properly expressed in Newtons, although kg is commonly used as well) that can be generated by a specific muscle or muscle group. Static or isometric strength can be conveniently measured using a variety of devices, including cable tensiometers and handgrip dynamometers. Unfortunately, measures of static strength are specific both to the muscle group and joint angle involved in testing and, therefore, their utility in describing overall muscular strength is limited. Peak force development in such tests is commonly referred to as the maximum voluntary contraction (MVC).

When testing involves movement of the body or an external load, then dynamic strength is being evaluated. The simplest measures of dynamic strength involve various 1-repetition maximum (1-RM; the heaviest weight that can be lifted only once) weight-lifting tests. After warm-up and familiarization with equipment, the subject is allowed up to five trials, with appropriate rest periods between, to achieve a 1-RM performance. Valid measures of general upper body strength include the 1-RM values for bench press or military press. Corresponding indices of lower body strength include 1-RM values for leg press or leg extension. If dynamic muscular performance tests involve maximum movement of the entire body within a short, nonfatiguing time frame (e.g., vertical jump), then muscular power is being evaluated. Normative tables for various strength tests are presented in Chapter 6.

Isokinetic testing involves the assessment of muscle tension generated throughout a range of joint motion at a constant angular velocity. Equipment which allows control of the speed of joint rotation (degrees/sec) as well as physical adjustability to test movement around various joints (e.g., knee, hip, shoulder, elbow) is available from several commercial sources. Such devices measure peak rotational force or torque, defined as "the measured ability of a rotation element to overcome turning resistance:"

torque (in Newton-meters or foot-pounds) = force × distance

An important drawback to such equipment is that it is extremely expensive compared to other strength-testing modalities.

MUSCULAR ENDURANCE

Muscular endurance is the ability of a muscle group to execute repeated contractions over a period of sufficient time duration to cause muscular fatigue, or to statically maintain a specific percentage of MVC for a prolonged period of time. Simple field tests such as the 60-second sit-up test or the maximum number of push-ups that can be performed without rest may be used to evaluate the endurance of the abdominal muscle groups and upper body muscles, respectively.[17,18] Methods of administration and age- and sex-specific percentile norms for these tests are available.[17,18] The sit-up test, however, has been criticized because of the involvement of accessory muscles (hip flexors) in addition to the abdominal muscles. Although scientific evidence is scarce, poor abdominal strength/endurance is commonly thought to contribute to muscular low back pain. Procedures for conducting a push-up muscular endurance test are given in Table 4–7.

Resistance training and isokinetic equipment can also be adapted to measure muscular endurance by selecting an appropriate submaximal level of resistance and measuring the number of repetitions or the duration of static contraction before fatigue. For example, the YMCA bench press test involves performing standardized repetitions at a rate of 30 repetitions /min. Men are tested using an 80-pound barbell and women using a 35-pound barbell. Subjects are scored by the number of successful repetitions.[18]

TABLE 4–7. PUSH-UP TEST PROCEDURES FOR MEASUREMENT OF MUSCULAR ENDURANCE

1. The push-up test is administered with male subjects in the standard "up" position (hands shoulder width apart, back straight, head up) and female subjects in the modified "knee push-up" position (ankles crossed, knees bent at 90° angle, back straight, hands shoulder width apart, head up)
2. When testing male subjects, the tester places a fist on the floor beneath the subject's chest and the subject must lower the body to the floor until the chest touches the tester's fist. The fist method is not used for female subjects, and no criteria are established for determining how much the torso must be lowered to count as a proper push-up
3. For both men and women, the subject's back must be straight at all times and the subject must push up to a straight arm position
4. The maximal number of push-ups performed consecutively without rest is counted as the score

FLEXIBILITY

Flexibility is the maximum ability to move a joint through a range of motion. It depends on a number of specific variables, including distensibility of the joint capsule, muscle temperature, muscle viscosity, etc. Additionally, compliance ("tightness") of various other tissues such as ligaments and tendons affects the range of motion. Like muscular strength, flexibility is specific. Therefore,

TABLE 4–8. TRUNK FLEXION (SIT-AND-REACH) TEST PROCEDURES*

1. Participant should perform a short warm-up prior to this test. It is also recommended that the participant refrain from fast, jerky movements which may increase the possibility of an injury. The participant's shoes should be removed
2. A yardstick is placed on the floor and tape placed across it at a right angle to the 15-inch mark. The participant sits with the yardstick between the legs, with legs extended at right angles to the taped line on the floor. Heels of the feet should touch the edge of the taped line and be about 10 to 12 inches apart. If a standard sit-and-reach box is available, heels should be placed against the edge of the box
3. The participant should slowly reach forward with both hands as far as possible on the yardstick, holding this position momentarily. Be sure that the participant keeps the hands parallel and does not lead with one hand. Fingertips can be overlapped and should be in contact with the yardstick or measuring portion of the sit-and-reach box
4. The score is the most distant point (in inches) reached on the yardstick with the fingertips. The best of three trials should be recorded. In order to assist with the best attempt, the participant should exhale and drop the head between the arms when reaching. Testers should ensure that the knees of the participant stay extended; however, the participant's knees should not be pressed down
5. The participant should breathe normally during the test and should not hold his/her breath at any time

*Adapted from Reference 18.

no single test can be generalized to evaluate total body flexibility. Laboratory tests usually quantify flexibility in terms of range of motion, expressed in degrees. Common devices for this purpose include various goniometers, electrogoniometers, and the Leighton flexometer. Field tests used for the evaluation of flexibility include the shoulder elevation test, ankle flexibility test, trunk flexion (sit-and-reach) test, and trunk extension test.

The trunk flexion or sit-and-reach test is often employed in health-oriented fitness evaluations to assess low back and hip flexibility. Poor lower back and hip flexibility may, in conjunction with poor abdominal strength/ endurance or other etiologic factors, contribute to development of muscular low back pain. This hypothesis, however, remains to be substantiated from a scientific perspective. Methods for administering this test are presented in Table 4–8. Normative data based on the testing of a large subject sample are presented in Chapter 6.

REFERENCES

1. Casperson CJ, Powell KE and Christenson GM: Physical activity, exercise and physical fitness: Definitions and distinctions for health-related research. *Public Health Reports* *100*:126–131, 1985.
2. Pate RR: The evolving definition of physical fitness. *Quest* *40*:174–179, 1988.
3. National Center for Health Statistics: *Health. United States, 1989.* Hyattsville, MD: Public Health Service [DHHS Publication No: (PHS) 90–1232], 1990.
4. Brozek J and Keys A: The evaluation of leanness-fatness in man: Norms and interrelationships. *Br J Nutr* *5*:194–206, 1951.
5. Wilmore J: Body composition in sports and exercise: Directions for future research. *Med Sci Sports Exerc* *15*:21–31, 1983.

6. Brozek J, Grande F, Anderson J, Keys A: Densitometric analysis of body composition: Revision of some quantitative assumptions. *Ann NY Acad Sci 110*:113–140, 1963.

7. Siri WE: Body composition from fluid spaces and density. *Univ Calif Donner Lab Med Phys Rep*, March 1956.

8. Jackson AS, Pollock, ML: Practical assessment of body composition. *Physician Sport Med 13*:76–90, 1985. (As published in: Nieman DC: The Sports Medicine Fitness Course, Bull Publ, Palo Alto, 1986, p. 101.)

9. Nieman DC: *Fitness and Your Health*. Palo Alto, CA: Bull Publishing Company, 1993, p. 74.

10. Jáequier E: Energy, obesity, and body weight standards. *Am J Clin Nutr 45*:1035–1047, 1987.

11. Van Itallie TB: Topography of body fat: Relationship to risk of cardiovascular and other diseases. In *Anthropometric Standardization Reference Manual*. Edited by TG Lohman, AF Roche and R Martorell: Champaign, IL: Human Kinetics Books, 1988.

12. Bray, GA and Gray DS: Obesity. Part 1—Pathogenesis. *Western J Med 149*:429–441, 1988.

13. Brodie DA: Techniques of measurement of body composition. *Sports Med 5*:11–40 and 74–98, 1988.

14. Noble BJ, Borg GAV, Jacobs I, Ceci R, Kaiser P: A category-ratio perceived exertion scale: Relationship to blood and muscle lactates and heart rate. *Med Sci Sports Exerc 15*:523–528, 1983.

15. Åstrand P-O and Ryhming I: A nomogram for calculation of aerobic capacity (physical fitness) from pulse rate during submaximal work. *J Appl Physiol 7*:218, 1954.

16. Åstrand I: Aerobic work capacity in men and women with special reference to age. *Acta Physiol Scand 49* (suppl. 169):45–60, 1960.

17. Gettman LR: Fitness Testing. In *Resource Manual for Guidelines for Exercise Testing and Prescription*. Edited by American College of Sports Medicine. Philadelphia: Lea & Febiger, 1989.

18. Golding LA, Myers CR and Sinning WE (eds.): *Y's Way to Physical Fitness*, 3rd ed. Champaign, IL: Human Kinetics Publishers, 1989.

chapter 5

CLINICAL EXERCISE TESTING

INDICATIONS AND APPLICATIONS

There are five general indications or applications for clinical exercise testing:

1. Pre-discharge Exercise Testing After Myocardial Infarction (MI)

Pre-discharge testing must be based on clinical assessment of the severity of the infarction, but has been performed in patients with uncomplicated infarction as soon as 3 days post-event.[1] Even maximal testing has been utilized safely by applying cautious termination criteria and careful patient selection, but in general a submaximal test to a predetermined heart rate or a rating of perceived exertion of 16–17 is adequate. This test can confirm that the patient is appropriately medicated to go home and reassure all concerned as to safe levels of activity during recuperation. In addition, in Q wave infarction patients, the hemodynamic responses may aid in identifying high-risk patients who may need further intervention or special monitoring during exercise.[2] In contrast, ST-segment responses are associated with increased risk in the non-Q wave MI patients.[3]

2. Post-Discharge Exercise Testing After MI, Percutaneous Transluminal Coronary Angioplasty (PTCA) or Coronary Artery Bypass Graft Surgery (CABG)

A maximal test can be performed when the patient is ready to return to full activities. The timing is typically about 3 weeks post-event but should be individualized. Exercise testing may be used to determine an appropriate exercise prescription for the patient, adjust medications, and determine if further interventions are required to lessen symptoms or improve prognosis.

3. Diagnostic Testing

Diagnostic testing is best utilized in patients with an intermediate probability of angiographically significant CAD as determined by symptoms (particularly atypical angina pectoris or dyspnea equivalent), ECG abnormalities, an exercise-related event, or possible history of a cardiac event. An intermediate probability rarely characterizes asymptomatic individuals even when multiple risk factors are present. In general, patients with a high probability of disease (i.e., typical angina, prior CABG, PTCA, or MI) are tested to assess residual ischemia and prognosis rather than for diagnostic purposes. While some groups are known to have a lower test specificity (women, individuals taking digoxin, and individuals with left ventricular hypertrophy and/or resting ST depression), sensitivity is not affected, so a standard exercise test remains the best initial diagnostic test.

4. Functional Testing

Maximal testing for the aim of establishing safe levels of exercise performance or for disability assessment can be done on any person, with or without heart disease. Aerobic capacity may be reported as the percentage of expected METs for age using a nomogram (Figure 5–1), with 100% being normal (separate nomograms are pro-

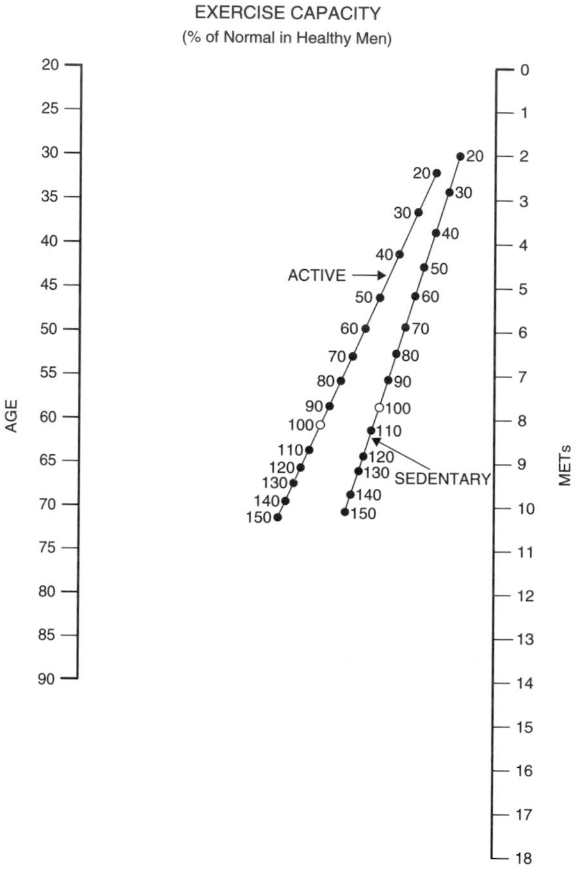

FIG. 5–1. Nomograms of percent normal exercise capacity in healthy men (this page) and in men referred for clinical testing (following page).

Continued on Next Page

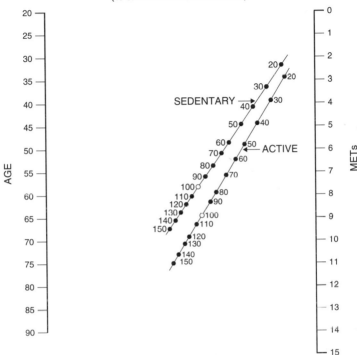

FIG. 5–1. *Continued*

vided for volunteers vs. referred subjects in keeping with the referenced source).[4]

5. Testing for Disease Severity and Prognosis

The magnitude of ischemia caused by a coronary lesion is directly proportional to the amount of ST depression, the number of ECG leads involved, and the duration of depression in recovery. It is inversely proportional to the ST slope, the double product at which the ST depression

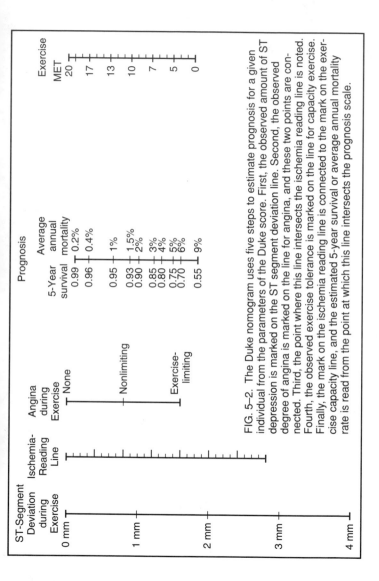

FIG. 5–2. The Duke nomogram uses five steps to estimate prognosis for a given individual from the parameters of the Duke score. First, the observed amount of ST segment deviation is marked on the ST segment deviation line. Second, the observed degree of angina is marked on the line for angina, and these two points are connected. Third, the point where this line intersects the ischemia reading line is noted. Fourth, the observed exercise tolerance is marked on the line for capacity exercise. Finally, the mark on the ischemia reading line is connected to the mark on the exercise capacity line, and the estimated 5-year survival or average annual mortality rate is read from the point at which this line intersects the prognosis scale.

occurs, and the maximal heart rate, systolic blood pressure, and MET level achieved. Since left ventricular function is more important than ischemia with respect to prognosis, exercise test responses linked to both LV function and ischemia such as maximal systolic blood pressure and METs are better indicators of prognosis. Clinically, this is reflected by the impact of congestive heart failure, which is associated with an annual mortality of 25%, in contrast to the 2% annual mortality in stable angina patients. Several numerical indices of prognosis have been published,[5,6] including the Duke nomogram[5] (Figure 5–2), which has been validated for the general population.

EXERCISE TEST MODALITIES

Three types of exercise can be used to stress the oxygen transport system: isometric, dynamic, and a combination of the two. Dynamic exercise is preferred to isometric exercise for testing since it can be graduated and controlled. It places a volume stress on the heart, however, rather than a pressure load. The cycle ergometer and the treadmill are the most commonly used dynamic exercise modalities. The former is less expensive, requires less space, and makes less noise. Electronically braked cycle ergometers maintain the work load over a wide range of pedaling speeds. In studies comparing upright cycle ergometer and treadmill exercise, maximal heart rate values have been demonstrated to be similar, whereas maximal oxygen uptake has been shown to be 10 to 15% greater during treadmill exercise.[7]

The treadmill should have a front rail and at least one side rail for patients to steady themselves. The patient should be told that he/she can hold on to the rails initially, but then should only use the rails for balance. A

FUNCTIONAL CLASS	CLINICAL STATUS	O₂ COST ml / kg / min	METS	BICYCLE ERGOMETER	TREADMILL PROTOCOLS		
						BRUCE	KATTUS
				1 WATT = 6 KP		3 MIN STAGES MPH \GR 5.5 20	
NORMAL AND I	HEALTHY, DEPENDENT ON AGE, ACTIVITY	56.0	16	FOR 70 KG BODY WEIGHT KP		5.0 18	
		52.5	15				MPH \GR
		49.0	14	1500			4 22
		45.5	13			4.2 16	
		42.0	12	1350			4 18
		38.5	11	1200			4 14
		35.0	10	1050		3.4 14	
	SEDENTARY HEALTHY	31.5	9	900			4 10
		28.0	8	750			
		24.5	7			2.5 12	3 10
II	LIMITED	21.0	6	600			2 10
	SYMPTOMATIC	17.5	5	450		1.7 10	
III		14.0	4	300		1.7 5	
		10.5	3	150			
		7.0	2			1.7 0	
IV		3.5	1				

FIG. 5–3. Common exercise protocols.

Continued on Next Page

small platform or stepping area at the level of the belt is advisable so that the patient can start the test by "pedaling" the belt with one foot prior to stepping on. An emergency stop button should be readily available for the staff only.

Arm ergometry is an alternative method of exercise testing for patients who cannot perform leg exercise.[8] Non-exercise cardiac stress pharmacologic techniques are currently more popular, however, and appear to offer increased sensitivity and specificity.

TREADMILL PROTOCOLS							METS
BALKE-WARE	**ELLESTAD**	**USAFSAM**	**"SLOW" USAFSAM**	**McHENRY**	**STANFORD**		
\GRADE AT 3.3 MPH 1-MIN STAGES	3/2/3 MIN STAGES				\GRADE AT 3 MPH	\GRADE AT 2 MPH	
	MPH | \GR	MPH | \GR	MPH | \GR	MPH | \GR			
26							
25	6 | 15						16
24		3.3 | 25					15
23							
22	5 | 15			MPH | \GR			14
21				3.3 | 21			
20		3.3 | 20					13
19				3.3 | 18			12
18					22.5		
17	5 | 10			3.3 | 15	20.0		11
16		3.3 | 15					
15			MPH | \GR		17.5		10
14			2 | 25				
13					15.0		9
12	4 | 10		2 | 20		12.5		8
11		3.3 | 101	2 | 15	3.3 | 12			
10	3 | 10				10.0	17.5	7
9				3.3 | 9			
8		3.3 | 5	2 | 10		7.5	14	6
7				3.3 | 6			
6	1.7 | 10				5.0	10.5	5
5			2 | 5				
4		3.3 | 0			2.5	7	4
3				2.0 | 3	0.0	3.5	3
2							2
1		2.0 | 0	2 | 0				1

FIG. 5–3. *Continued*

EXERCISE PROTOCOLS

The most common exercise protocols and the predicted VO_2 for each stage are illustrated in Figure 5–3. The Bruce protocol remains the most commonly used protocol; however, it employs relatively large and unequal increments (i.e., METs/stage) every 3 minutes. Such increments have been shown to overestimate exercise capacity. Protocols with larger increments (i.e., Bruce, Ellestad) are better suited for screening younger and/or active individuals while protocols with smaller increments (i.e., Naughton,

Balke-Ware, USAFSAM) are best for older or deconditioned individuals and patients with cardiovascular or respiratory disease. An alternative approach to incremental exercise testing which has gained popularity in recent years is the ramp protocol, in which work increases at a constant and continuous rate.[9]

Whichever exercise protocol is chosen, it should be individualized; e.g., treadmill speed should be established based on the individual's capabilities. Increments in work load should be chosen such that the total test time should ideally be 8 to 12 minutes.[10] For example, increments of 10 to 15 W/min can be used on the cycle ergometer for elderly persons, deconditioned individuals, and patients with disease. Increases in grade of 1 to 3% per minute can be used for treadmill tests for these same populations.

MEASUREMENTS

HEART RATE AND BLOOD PRESSURE

Heart rate (HR) and blood pressure (BP) must be measured prior to, during, and following the graded exercise test. Table 5–1 indicates the frequency and sequence of these measures. It is important that a standardized procedure be adopted for each laboratory so that baseline measures can be assessed more accurately when repeat testing is performed.

Though numerous devices have been developed to automate blood pressure measurement during exercise, none can be recommended unequivocally at the present time. Mercury manometers are favored over anaeroid manometers, which require frequent and more difficult calibration. Tables 5–2 and 5–3 suggest methods for assessment and potential sources of error. If systolic blood pressure appears to be decreasing with increasing

TABLE 5–1. SEQUENCE OF MEASURES FOR HEART RATE, BLOOD PRESSURE, AND ELECTROCARDIOGRAM DURING EXERCISE TESTING

Pre-Test

1. 12-lead ECG in supine and exercise postures
2. BP supine and in the exercise posture

Exercise

1. 12-lead ECG recorded during last minute of every stage or every 3 minutes (observed every minute on monitor)
2. BP during last minute of each stage
3. Rating scales: RPE at the end of each stage, other scales if applicable

In addition, all of the above should be assessed and recorded whenever symptoms or ECG changes occur.

Post-Test

1. 12-lead ECG immediately post exercise, then every 1 to 2 minutes for at least 5 minutes or longer to allow any exercise-induced changes to return to baseline
2. BP immediately post exercise, then every 1 to 2 minutes until stabilized near baseline level
3. Symptomatic ratings using appropriate scales for as long as symptoms persist post exercise

TABLE 5–2. PROCEDURES FOR ASSESSMENT OF BLOOD PRESSURE AT REST

1. Subject seated for at least 5 minutes with elbow slightly flexed
2. Wrap cuff firmly around upper arm at heart level; align cuff with brachial artery
3. Place stethoscope bell below the antecubital space over brachial artery
4. Quickly inflate cuff pressure to 200 mm Hg or 20 mm Hg above estimated systolic BP
5. Slowly release pressure at rate equal to 2 to 3 mm Hg/sec, noting first Korotkoff sound
6. Continue releasing pressure, noting when sound becomes muffled (4th phase diastolic BP) and when sound disappears (5th phase diastolic BP).

TABLE 5–3. POTENTIAL SOURCES OF ERROR IN BLOOD
PRESSURE ASSESSMENT

1. Inaccurate sphygmomanometer
2. Improper cuff size
3. Auditory acuity of technician
4. Rate of inflation or deflation of cuff pressure
5. Experience of technician
6. Reaction time of technician
7. Improper stethoscope placement or pressure
8. Background noise
9. Allowing patient to hold treadmill handrails
10. Certain physiological abnormalities, e.g., damaged brachial
    artery, subclavian steal syndrome, a-v fistula

intensity, it should be taken again immediately.[11] If a
drop in systolic blood pressure of 20 mm Hg or more
occurs, or if it drops below the value obtained in the
standing position prior to testing, the test should be
stopped, particularly if accompanied by signs or symptoms (see Table 5–4 for Test Termination criteria).

EXPIRED GASES

Because of the inaccuracies associated with estimating
oxygen consumption and METs from work rate (i.e.,
treadmill speed and grade), many laboratories directly
measure expired gases. Measurement of expired gases is
not necessary for clinical exercise testing, but the additional information provides important physiological data
(e.g., ventilation, ventilatory threshold, and respiratory
exchange ratio).

ELECTROCARDIOGRAPHIC (ECG) MONITORING

Proper skin preparation is essential for recording the electrocardiogram during an exercise test. It is important to
lower the resistance at the skin-electrode interface and

TABLE 5–4. ABSOLUTE AND RELATIVE INDICATIONS FOR
TERMINATION OF AN EXERCISE TEST

Absolute Indications

1. Acute myocardial infarction or suspicion of a myocardial infarction
2. Onset of moderate-to-severe angina
3. Drop in SBP with increasing workload accompanied by signs or symptoms or drop below standing resting pressure
4. Serious arrhythmias (e.g., second- or third-degree atrioventricular block, sustained ventricular tachycardia or increasing premature ventricular contractions, atrial fibrillation with fast ventricular response)
5. Signs of poor perfusion, including pallor, cyanosis, or cold and clammy skin
6. Unusual or severe shortness of breath
7. Central nervous system symptoms, including ataxia, vertigo, visual or gait problems, or confusion
8. Technical inability to monitor the ECG
9. Patient's request

Relative Indications

1. Pronounced ECG changes from baseline [>2mm of horizontal or downsloping ST-segment depression, or >2mm of ST-segment elevation (except in aVR)]
2. Any chest pain that is increasing
3. Physical or verbal manifestations of severe fatigue or shortness of breath
4. Wheezing
5. Leg cramps or intermittent claudication (grade 3 on 4-point scale)
6. Hypertensive response (SBP >260 mm Hg; DBP >115 mm Hg)
7. Less serious arrhythmias such as supraventricular tachycardia
8. Exercise-induced bundle branch block that cannot be distinguished from ventricular tachycardia

thereby improve the signal-to-noise ratio. The general areas for electrode placement are shaved if hair is present and cleansed with an alcohol-saturated gauze pad. The next step is to remove the superficial layer of skin using light abrasion with fine-grain emery paper or gauze. The electrodes are placed using anatomic landmarks (see

Appendix C) that are most easily located with the patient supine.

Bipolar lead systems have been used historically because of the relatively short time required for placement, the relative freedom from motion artifact, and the ease with which noise problems can be located. Clinically, bipolar leads have been replaced by the routine monitoring of 12 leads. Since electrodes placed on wrists and ankles obstruct exercise, these electrodes are placed on the torso at the base of the limbs for exercise testing.[12] Since torso leads may give a slightly different ECG configuration when compared to the standard 12-lead resting ECG, use of torso leads should be noted on the ECG.

Signal processing techniques have made it possible to average ECG waveforms and to remove noise, but caution is urged since signal averaging can actually distort the signal.[13] Moreover, most manufacturers do not specify how such procedures modify the ECG. It is therefore important to consider the raw ECG data first, using the filtered data to aid interpretation if no distortion is obvious.

SUBJECTIVE RATINGS

The measurement of perceptual responses during exercise testing can provide useful clinical information. Somatic ratings of perceived exertion (RPE) and/or specific symptomatic complaints (degree of chest pain, burning, discomfort, etc., dyspnea, or leg discomfort/pain) should be routinely assessed during clinical exercise tests. The patient is asked to provide subjective estimates during the last 15 seconds of each exercise intensity by either verbal or manual methods. For example, the individual can provide a number verbally or point to a number if a mouthpiece or face mask is being used. The exercise technician should state the number out loud to confirm the correct rating.

Either the 6 to 20 or the 0 to 10 (see Chapter 4) category ratio scales may be used for RPE during exercise testing. Prior to the start of the exercise test the patient should be given clear and concise instructions for use of the selected scale. The following written statements are an example of instructions for use of the 0 to 10 category scale:

"This is a scale for rating perceived exertion. Perceived exertion is the overall effort or distress of your body during exercise. The number 0 represents no perceived exertion or leg discomfort and the number 10 represents the greatest amount of exertion that you have ever experienced. At various times during the exercise test you will be asked to point to a number which indicates your rating of perceived exertion at the time. One of the technicians will say the number out loud in order to make sure that we understand your selection. Do you have any questions?"

The 6 to 20 category scale has a history of extensive use in clinical exercise testing. In 1982, this scale was revised into a 0 to 10 category scale with ratio properties based on descriptors positioned alongside specific numbers. Although the 0 to 10 scale has theoretical advantages over the 6 to 20 scale, either instrument can be used to obtain RPE ratings.

When subjects become symptomatic during exercise, use of alternative rating scales which are specific to symptomatology are recommended. A frequently used scale for assessment of angina is:

1+	Light, barely noticeable
2+	Moderate, bothersome
3+	Severe, very uncomfortable
4+	Most severe or intense pain ever experienced

POST-EXERCISE PERIOD

If maximal sensitivity is to be achieved with an exercise test, patients should be supine during the post-exercise period,[14] although it is advantageous to record about 10 seconds of electrocardiographic data while the patient is in the upright position immediately post-exercise. Having the patient perform a cool-down walk after the test may decrease the risk of hypotension but can attenuate the magnitude of ST-segment depression. When the test is being performed for non-diagnostic purposes, an active cool-down is usually preferable, e.g., slow walking (1.0 to 1.5 mph) or continued cycling against minimal resistance. Monitoring should continue for at least 6 to 8 minutes after exercise or until ECG changes return to baseline. ST-segment changes which occur only during the post-exercise period are not likely to be false-positives. In patients who are severely dyspneic, the supine posture may exacerbate the condition and sitting may be a more appropriate posture.

INDICATIONS FOR EXERCISE TEST TERMINATION

The absolute and relative indications for termination of an exercise test are listed in Table 5–4. Absolute indications are clear-cut, whereas relative indications may sometimes be re-evaluated when sound clinical judgment supersedes the stated criteria.

Complications associated with exercise testing can often be avoided by having an experienced professional standing next to the patient, measuring BP and assessing patient status. In most instances, a symptom-limited maximal test is preferred; in some patients considered to be at high risk because of clinical data, it may be appropriate to stop at a submaximal level. If the measurement of maximal exercise capacity or other information is needed, it is better to repeat the test on a subsequent day, once the patient has demonstrated safe performance of a submaximal work load.

RADIONUCLIDE EXERCISE TESTING

There are two basic types of radionuclide exercise testing currently available: myocardial perfusion imaging (using thallium or technetium-tagged isonitriles) and radionuclide ventriculography [using the first pass or computer averaged (MUGA) methods of observing the passage of technetium-tagged red cells through the heart].[19] Perfusion imaging has advantages in terms of sensitivity and specificity compared with the standard exercise ECG; consequently, it is the first additional test when the standard exercise test is equivocal or incongruous with respect to other clinical findings or symptoms. The recent addition of three-dimensional imaging (SPECT) has improved the specificity of perfusion imaging. It also permits the localization of ischemia to a coronary artery distribution, which is not possible with the standard exercise test. Finally, thallium tests allow for the differentiation of fixed (infarct) versus reversible (ischemia, injury) defects. Radionuclide ventriculography permits the assessment of ventricular function (in particular, ejection fraction) during cycle ergometry; however, the specificity of the ejection fraction responses has been poor and this test is rarely used for diagnosing CAD.

NON-EXERCISE STRESS TESTS OR PHARMACOLOGICAL TESTS

The two most commonly used pharmacological tests are dipyridamole (Persantine) perfusion imaging (using thallium or isonitriles) and dobutamine (or arbutamine) echocardiography. These non-exercise tests have excellent characteristics for diagnosing coronary artery disease and evaluating its severity. They are indicated for patients who cannot exercise due to peripheral vascular disease, neurological or muscular disease or disability due to other diseases, or in patients who are unable to achieve an adequate work rate during a standard exercise test. Dipyridamole infusion results in vasodilation of normal coronary arteries with little impact on obstructive lesions. The difference in blood flow between normal and obstructed coronary arteries is visualized. Dobutamine and other chronotropic agents increase heart rate and myocardial oxygen demand and elicit wall motion abnormalities that can be visualized by the echocardiogram. ECG changes during these procedures are not very sensitive, but are highly specific for CAD.

CONSIDERATIONS FOR PULMONARY PATIENTS

The vast majority of patients with chronic respiratory disease [e.g., asthma, chronic obstructive pulmonary disease (COPD), and interstitial lung disease] seek medical attention because of exertional dyspnea or breathlessness. The medical history should include questions that address the characteristics of breathlessness, including descriptive qualities, onset, frequency, severity, and activities and triggers that provoke dyspnea. This information should be used by the health care provider to consider possible diagnoses and to clarify the impact that breathlessness has on an individual's functional status. Any one of many temporally related events (e.g., weight gain, respiratory infection, and new medication) might explain the likely cause of breathlessness.

In addition, it may be helpful for the health care provider to quantify the severity of dyspnea as part of the medical history. Various indirect scales or questionnaires have been developed to measure dyspnea intensity. Two such scales are the Baseline (BDI) and Transition (TDI) Dyspnea Indexes,[16] which incorporate three components (task, effort, and function) that influence dyspnea (Table 5–5). Scores for baseline and transition ratings of dyspnea

TABLE 5–5. DYSPNEA INDEXES

Baseline Dyspnea Index (BDI)

Component	Grades
Functional impairment	0 to 4
Magnitude of task	0 to 4
Magnitude of effort	0 to 4
BDI Focal Score	0 to 12

Transition Dyspnea Index (TDI)

Component	Grades
*Change in functional impairment	−3 to +3
*Change in magnitude of task	−3 to +3
*Change in magnitude of effort	−3 to +3
TDI Focal Score	−9 to +9

*Change from baseline state.

are obtained through an interview by a professional experienced in obtaining a clinical history for pulmonary disease. For each category, the interviewer asks open-ended questions about the patient's experience of breathlessness, while at the same time focusing on specific criteria for evaluating the intensity of dyspnea. Based on the patient's responses, the interviewer can grade the degree of impairment related to dyspnea.

Another useful scale is the dyspnea component of the Chronic Respiratory Questionnaire (CRQ)[17] which considers the five most bothersome activities for the individual that cause exertional breathlessness (Table 5–6). A list of 26 activities is read to the patient who responds whether shortness of breath occurred during that activity. After the patient determines the five most common dyspnea-causing activities, the severity of breathlessness is graded on a scale of 1 ("extremely short of breath") to 7 ("not at all short of breath"). These scores are added to obtain an

TABLE 5–6. DYSPNEA COMPONENT OF CHRONIC RESPIRATORY DISEASE QUESTIONNAIRE (CRQ)

A. Patient determines 5 most important activities that cause dyspnea and affect daily life by:
 1. self-selection
 2. review of a list of 26 activities
B. For each activity, severity of dyspnea is measured using a 1 ("extremely short of breath") to 7 ("not at all short of breath") scale

Activity	Score
A	1 to 7
B	1 to 7
C	1 to 7
D	1 to 7
E	1 to 7
CRQ dyspnea score	5 to 35

overall CRQ score ranging from 5 to 35. Both the BDI/TDI and the dyspnea scale of the CRQ have been shown to be valid, reliable, and responsive instruments.[18]

LUNG FUNCTION

Detailed information on selection and interpretation of lung function tests is provided in Chapter 3. The measured maximal voluntary ventilation (MVV) or $FEV_{1.0} \times 35$ (or 40) can be used as an estimate of the predicted maximal exercise ventilation ($\dot{V}_{Emax}$).[19,20]

EXERCISE TESTING OF PULMONARY PATIENTS

Exercise testing can be helpful for differentiating exertional breathlessness secondary to lung or cardiac diseases. Indications for cardiopulmonary exercise testing in pulmonary patients are:

- Cause of breathlessness remains unclear despite results from pulmonary function tests
- Patient's severity of breathlessness is disproportionate to objective data
- Both cardiac and respiratory diseases coexist
- Deconditioning, physiological factors (e.g., anxiety), or obesity are suspected causes for exertional dyspnea
- To evaluate for exercise-induced oxygen desaturation
- Exercise prescription

Although COPD is diagnosed by history and pulmonary function tests, spirometry estimates a patient's ventilatory capacity (but not the ventilatory requirements for exertional activities). Furthermore, many patients with COPD have concomitant coronary artery disease, deconditioning, or anxiety/depression that might also reduce exercise performance. Exercise testing can provide important clinical data about these and other possible conditions that might cause dyspnea and/or limit exercise performance in patients with COPD.

Measurement of ventilation is essential in exercise testing of patients with pulmonary disease. Relatively inexpensive flowmeters can be used. On the other hand, it is clearly preferable to also measure components of $\dot{V}_E$, frequency of respiration and tidal volume, as well as expired gases, $\dot{V}O_2$ and $\dot{V}CO_2$.

It is also important to measure gas exchange in pulmonary patients because oxygen desaturation may occur during exertion. Although measurement of P_aO_2 and P_aCO_2 from arterial blood has been the standard in the past, the availability of noninvasive oximeters has generally replaced the need to routinely draw arterial blood in most patients. In patients with pulmonary disease, measurements of oxygen saturation (S_aO_2) from oximetry at rest correlate reasonably well with S_aO_2 measured from arterial blood (95% confidence limits are ±3 to 5% saturation).[21] Carboxyhemoglobin (COHb) levels greater than 4% and black skin may adversely affect the accuracy of pulse oximeters,[22,23] and most oximeters are inaccurate at an $S_aO_2 \leq 85\%$.

As previously discussed, it is important to measure perceptual responses during exercise in patients with respiratory disease. The 6 to 20 and 0 to 10 RPE scales[24] are commonly used.

SUMMARY OF METHODOLOGY

Testing procedures for pulmonary patients are similar to those described for cardiac patients. Preparing the pulmonary patient physically and emotionally for testing is critical. A brief physical exam is always necessary to rule out nonpulmonary diseases. The exercise test protocol should be progressive, with even increments in speed and grade whenever possible. Smaller and more frequent work increments are preferable to larger and less frequent increases. The value of individualizing the exercise protocol, rather than using the same protocol for every patient, has been emphasized by many investigators. The optimal test duration is from 8 to 12 minutes. The protocol work loads should be adjusted to permit this estimation of exercise capacity, and can be individualized for every patient to yield a targeted test duration.

REFERENCES

1. Topol EJ, Burek K, O'Neill WW, et al.: A randomized controlled trial of hospital discharge three days after myocardial infarction in the era of reperfusion. *N Engl J Med* *318*:1083–1088, 1988.
2. Froelicher VF, Perdue S, Powen W, et al.: Application of meta-analysis using an electronic spread sheet to exercise testing in patients after myocardial infarction. *Am J Med* *83*:1045–1052, 1987.
3. Klein J, Froelicher VF, Detrano R, et al.: Does the rest electrocardiogram after myocardial infarction determine the predictive value of exercise-induced ST depression? A 2 year follow-up study in a veteran population. *J Am Coll Cardiol* *14*:305–311, 1989.
4. Morris CK, Myers JN, Froelicher VF, et al.: Nomogram based on metabolic equivalents and age for assessing aerobic exercise capacity in men. *J Am Coll Cardiol 22*:175–182, 1993.
5. Mark DB, Shaw L, Harrell FE, et al.: Prognostic value of a treadmill exercise score in outpatients with suspected coronary artery disease. *N Engl J Med* 325:849–853, 1991.
6. Froelicher VF, Morrow K, Brown M, et al.: Prediction of atherosclerotic cardiovascular death in men using a prognostic score. *Am J Cardiol 73*:133–138, 1994.

7. Myers J, Buchanan N, Walsh D, et al.: Comparison of the ramp versus standard exercise protocols. *J Am Coll Cardiol* 17:1334–1342, 1991.

8. Balady GJ, Weiner DA, McCabe CH, et al.: Value of arm exercise testing in detecting coronary artery disease. *Am J Cardiol* 55:37–39, 1985.

9. Myers J, Buchanan N, Smith D, et al.: Individualized ramp treadmill: Observations on a new protocol. *Chest* 101: 2305–2315, 1992.

10. Buchfuhrer MJ, Hansen JE, Robinson TE, et al.: Optimizing the exercise protocol for cardiopulmonary assessment. *J Appl Physiol* 55:1558–1564, 1983.

11. Dubach P, Froelicher VF, Klein J, et al.: Exercise-induced hypotension in a male population—criteria, causes, and prognosis. *Circulation* 78:1380–1387, 1989.

12. Gamble P, McManus H, Jensen D, et al.: A comparison of the standard 12-lead electrocardiogram to exercise electrode placements. *Chest* 85:616–622, 1984.

13. Milliken JA, Abdollah H, Burgraf GW: False-positive treadmill exercise tests due to computer signal averaging. *Am J Cardiol* 65:946–948, 1990.

14. Lachterman B, Lehmann KG, Abrahamson D, Froelicher VF: "Recovery only" ST segment depression and the predictive accuracy of the exercise test. *Ann Intern Med* 112:11–16, 1990.

15. Froelicher VF, Myers JM, Follansbee WP, et al.: Stress radionuclide myocardial perfusion imaging. In *Exercise and the Heart, Third Edition,* Missouri: Mosby, 1993.

16. Mahler DA, Weinberg DH, Wells CK, and Feinstein AR: The measurement of dyspnea: Contents, interobserver agreement, and physiologic correlates of two new clinical indexes. *Chest* 85:751–758, 1984.

17. Guyatt GH, Berman LB, Townsend M, Pugsley SO, Chambers LW: A measure of quality of life for clinical trials in chronic lung disease. *Thorax* 42:773–778, 1987.

18. Mahler DA, Horner A: Clinical measurement of dyspnea. In *Dyspnea,* Edited by DA Mahler. Mt. Kisco, NY: Futura Publishing Co., Inc., 1990.

19. Wasserman K, Hansen JE, Sue DY, Whipp B: *Principles of Exercise Testing and Interpretation.* Philadelphia: Lea & Febiger, 1987.

20. Jones NL: *Clinical Exercise Testing.* Philadelphia: WB Saunders, 1988.

21. Ries AL, Farrow JT, Clausen JL: Accuracy of two ear oximeters at rest and during exercise in pulmonary patients. *Am Rev Respir Dis 132*:685–689, 1985.
22. Zeballos RJ, Weisman IM: Reliability of noninvasive oximetry in black subjects during exercise and hypoxia. *Am Rev Respir Dis 144*:1240–1244, 1991.
23. Orenstein DM, Curtis SE, Nixon PA, Hartigan ER: Accuracy of three pulse oximeters during exercise and hypoxemia in patients with cystic fibrosis. *Chest 104*:1187–1190, 1993.
24. Borg GAV: Psychophysical bases of perceived exertion. *Med Sci Sports Exerc 14*:377–381, 1982.

chapter 6

INTERPRETATION OF TEST DATA

INTERPRETATION OF FITNESS TEST DATA

Results from the various fitness tests described in Chapter 4 may be utilized in various ways. For example, serial testing allows for intra-individual comparisons of test results, which in turn provides a direct means of demonstrating changes in fitness that may result from training or detraining. On the other hand, it is often desirable to interpret test results with respect to external data. There is a distinct difference between *standards* and *normative data (or "norms")*. The latter are based on normal distributions of data collected from large subject samples, and are typically stratified by age and gender. The former refers to threshold values which have been validated as meaningful positive or negative indicators of risk for disease or other untoward event.

A wide range of acceptable fitness values exist, and multiple factors (e.g., medical and health history, family history, risk profiles, etc.) must be considered when interpreting such information. Tables 6–1 through 6–14 present normative data for all of the health-related fitness components for men and women of various ages, provided by the Institute for Aerobics Research in Dallas, TX.[1]

TABLE 6–1. BODY COMPOSITION (% BODY FAT) FOR MEN*

%	Age					
	20–29	30–39	40–49	50–59	60+	
99	2.4	5.2	6.6	8.8	7.7	
95	5.2	9.1	11.4	12.9	13.1	S
90	7.1	11.3	13.6	15.3	15.3	
85	8.3	12.7	15.1	16.9	17.2	
80	9.4	13.9	16.3	17.9	18.4	E
75	10.6	14.9	17.3	19.0	19.3	
70	11.8	15.9	18.1	19.8	20.3	
65	12.9	16.6	18.8	20.6	21.1	
60	14.1	17.5	19.6	21.3	22.0	G
55	15.0	18.2	20.3	22.1	22.6	
50	15.9	19.0	21.1	22.7	23.5	
45	16.8	19.7	21.8	23.4	24.3	
40	17.4	20.5	22.5	24.1	25.0	F
35	18.3	21.4	23.3	24.9	25.9	
30	19.5	22.3	24.1	25.7	26.7	
25	20.7	23.2	25.0	26.6	27.6	
20	22.4	24.2	26.1	27.5	28.5	P
15	23.9	25.5	27.3	28.8	29.7	
10	25.9	27.3	28.9	30.3	31.2	
5	29.1	29.9	31.5	32.4	33.4	VP
1	36.4	35.6	37.4	38.1	41.3	
N =	1342	5611	5724	3275	984	
TOTAL N = 16936						

*Data provided by the Institute for Aerobics Research, Dallas, TX (1994).
S, superior; E, excellent; G, good; F, fair; P, poor; VP, very poor.

TABLE 6–2. BODY COMPOSITION (% BODY FAT) FOR WOMEN*

%	Age					
	20–29	30–39	40–49	50–59	60+	
99	5.4	7.3	11.6	11.6	15.4	
95	10.8	13.4	16.1	18.8	16.8	S
90	14.5	15.5	18.5	21.6	21.1	
85	16.0	16.9	20.3	23.6	23.5	
80	17.1	18.0	21.3	25.0	25.1	E
75	18.2	19.1	22.4	25.8	26.7	
70	19.0	20.0	23.5	26.6	27.5	
65	19.8	20.8	24.3	27.4	28.5	
60	20.6	21.6	24.9	28.5	29.3	G
55	21.3	22.4	25.5	29.2	29.9	
50	22.1	23.1	26.4	30.1	30.9	
45	22.7	24.0	27.3	30.8	31.8	
40	23.7	24.9	28.1	31.6	32.5	F
35	24.4	26.0	29.0	32.6	33.0	
30	25.4	27.0	30.1	33.5	34.3	
25	26.6	28.1	31.1	34.3	35.5	
20	27.7	29.3	32.1	35.6	36.6	P
15	29.8	31.0	33.3	36.6	38.0	
10	32.1	32.8	35.0	37.9	39.3	
5	35.4	35.7	37.8	39.6	40.5	VP
1	40.5	40.0	45.5	50.8	47.0	
N =	638	1336	1175	708	250	
TOTAL N = 4107						

*Data provided by the Institute for Aerobics Research, Dallas, TX (1994).
S, superior; E, excellent; G, good; F, fair; P, poor; VP, very poor.

GRADED EXERCISE TESTING AS A SCREENING TOOL FOR CORONARY ARTERY DISEASE

Recent data convincingly demonstrate the inappropriateness of including graded exercise testing (GXT) as part of routine health screening in apparently healthy individuals. When 195 individuals who demonstrated significant

TABLE 6-3. AEROBIC POWER TESTS (MEN)*

%	Age 20-29 Balke Treadmill (time)	$\dot{V}O_2$ Max (ml/kg/min)	12 Min Run Distance (miles)	1.5 Mile Run (time)	Age 30-39 Balke Treadmill (time)	$\dot{V}O_2$ Max (ml/kg/min)	12 Min Run Distance (miles)	1.5 Mile Run (time)	
99	30:20	58.79	1.94	7:29	29:00	58.86	1.89	7:11	S
95	27:00	53.97	1.81	8:13	26:00	52.53	1.77	8:44	
90	25:11	51.35	1.74	9:09	24:30	50.36	1.71	9:30	
85	24:00	49.64	1.69	9:45	23:00	48.20	1.65	10:16	
80	23:00	48.20	1.65	10:16	22:00	46.75	1.61	10:47	E
75	22:10	46.99	1.62	10:42	21:00	45.31	1.57	11:18	
70	22:00	46.75	1.61	10:47	20:30	44.59	1.55	11:34	
65	21:00	45.31	1.57	11:18	20:00	43.87	1.53	11:49	
60	20:15	44.23	1.54	11:41	19:00	42.42	1.49	12:20	G
55	20:00	43.87	1.53	11:49	18:25	41.58	1.47	12:38	
50	19:03	42.49	1.50	12:18	18:00	40.98	1.45	12:51	
45	19:00	42.42	1.49	12:20	17:00	39.53	1.41	13:22	
40	18:00	40.98	1.45	12:51	16:32	38.86	1.39	13:36	F
35	17:30	40.26	1.43	13:06	16:00	38.09	1.37	13:53	
30	17:00	39.53	1.41	13:22	15:30	37.37	1.35	14:08	
25	16:00	38.09	1.37	13:53	15:00	36.65	1.33	14:24	
20	15:20	37.13	1.34	14:13	14:06	35.35	1.29	14:52	P
15	15:00	36.65	1.33	14:24	13:10	34.00	1.25	15:20	
10	13:30	34.48	1.27	15:10	12:09	32.53	1.21	15:52	
5	11:30	31.57	1.19	16:12	11:00	30.87	1.17	16:27	VP
1	8:23	27.05	1.06	17:48	8:00	26.54	1.13	18:00	

N = 1675   N = 7094

Continued on Next Page

113

TABLE 6-3. Continued

%	Balke Treadmill (time)	V̇O₂ Max (ml/kg/min)	12 Min Run Distance (miles)	1.5 Mile Run (time)	Balke Treadmill (time)	V̇O₂ Max (ml/kg/min)	12 Min Run Distance (miles)	1.5 Mile Run (time)	
	Age 40–49				**Age 50–59**				
99	28:00	55.42	1.85	7:42	26:00	52.53	1.77	8:44	
95	24:30	50.36	1.71	9:30	22:15	47.11	1.62	10:40	S
90	23:00	48.20	1.65	10:16	21:00	45.31	1.57	11:18	
85	21:00	45.31	1.57	11:18	19:00	42.42	1.49	12:20	
80	20:10	44.11	1.54	11:44	18:00	40.98	1.45	12:51	E
75	20:00	43.89	1.53	11:49	17:00	39.53	1.41	13:22	
70	18:32	41.75	1.47	12:34	16:15	38.45	1.38	13:45	
65	18:00	40.98	1.45	12:51	15:40	37.61	1.35	14:03	
60	17:15	39.89	1.42	13:14	15:00	36.65	1.33	14:24	G
55	17:00	39.53	1.41	13:22	14:30	36.10	1.31	14:40	
50	16:00	38.09	1.37	13:53	14:00	35.20	1.29	14:55	
45	15:30	37.37	1.35	14:08	13:15	34.12	1.26	15:08	
40	15:00	36.69	1.33	14:29	13:00	33.76	1.25	15:26	F
35	14:15	35.56	1.30	14:47	12:07	32.48	1.22	15:53	
30	13:57	35.13	1.29	14:56	12:00	32.31	1.21	15:57	
25	13:00	33.76	1.25	15:26	11:08	31.06	1.17	16:23	
20	12:30	33.04	1.23	15:41	10:30	30.15	1.15	16:43	P
15	12:00	32.31	1.21	15:57	10:00	29.43	1.13	16:58	
10	10:59	30.85	1.17	16:28	9:00	27.98	1.09	17:29	
5	6:21	28.29	1.10	17:23	7:00	25.09	1.01	18:31	VP
1	6:21	24.15	.98	18:51	4:54	22.06	.92	19:36	
	N = 6837				N = 3808				

Continued on Next Page

114

TABLE 6–3. Continued

			Age 60+		
%	Balke Treadmill (time)	$\dot{V}O_{2\,Max}$ (ml/kg/min)	12 Min Run Distance (miles)	1.5 Mile Run (time)	
99	24:29	50.39	1.71	9:30	S
95	20:56	45.21	1.57	11:20	
90	19:00	42.46	1.49	12:20	
85	17:00	39.53	1.41	13:22	
80	16:00	38.09	1.37	13:53	E
75	15:00	36.65	1.30	14:24	
70	14:04	35.30	1.29	14:53	
65	13:22	39.29	1.26	15:19	
60	12:53	33.59	1.24	15:29	G
55	12:03	32.39	1.21	15:55	
50	11:40	31.83	1.19	16:07	
45	11:00	30.87	1.17	16:27	
40	10:30	30.15	1.15	16:43	F
35	10:00	29.43	1.13	16:58	
30	9:30	28.70	1.11	17:14	
25	8:54	27.89	1.08	17:32	
20	8:00	26.54	1.05	18:00	P
15	7:00	25.05	1.01	18:31	
10	5:35	23.05	.95	19:15	
5	4:00	20.76	.89	20:04	VP
1	2:17	18.26	.82	20:57	

N = 1005

*Data provided by the Institute for Aerobics Research, Dallas, TX (1994). S, superior; E, excellent; G, good; F, fair; P, poor; VP, very poor.

115

TABLE 6-4. AEROBIC POWER TESTS (WOMEN)*

%	Age 20–29 Balke Treadmill (time)	V̇O₂ Max (ml/kg/min)	12 Min Run Distance (miles)	1.5 Mile Run (time)	Age 30–39 Balke Treadmill (time)	V̇O₂ Max (ml/kg/min)	12 Min Run Distance (miles)	1.5 Mile Run (time)	
99	26:21	53.03	1.78	8:33	23:22	48.73	1.66	10:05	
95	22:00	46.75	1.61	10:47	20:00	43.87	1.53	11:49	S
90	20:12	44.15	1.54	11:43	18:00	40.98	1.45	12:51	
85	19:00	42.42	1.49	12:20	17:30	40.26	1.43	13:06	
80	18:00	40.98	1.45	12:51	16:20	38.57	1.38	13:43	E
75	17:00	39.53	1.41	13:22	15:30	37.37	1.35	14:08	
70	16:00	38.09	1.37	13:53	15:00	36.65	1.33	14:24	
65	15:30	37.37	1.35	14:08	14:10	35.44	1.29	14:50	
60	15:00	36.65	1.33	14:24	13:35	34.60	1.27	15:08	G
55	14:39	36.14	1.31	14:35	13:10	33.85	1.26	15:20	
50	14:00	35.20	1.29	14:55	13:00	33.76	1.25	15:26	
45	13:30	34.48	1.27	15:10	12:10	32.41	1.22	15:47	
40	13:00	33.76	1.25	15:26	12:00	32.31	1.21	15:57	F
35	12:17	32.72	1.22	15:48	11:09	31.09	1.17	16:23	
30	12:00	32.31	1.21	15:57	10:45	30.51	1.16	16:35	
25	11:03	30.94	1.17	16:26	10:00	29.93	1.13	16:58	
20	10:50	30.63	1.16	16:33	9:30	28.70	1.11	17:14	P
15	10:00	29.43	1.13	16:58	9:00	27.98	1.09	17:29	
10	9:17	28.39	1.10	17:21	8:00	26.54	1.05	18:00	
5	7:33	25.89	1.03	18:14	7:00	25.09	1.01	18:31	VP
1	5:15	22.57	.94	19:25	5:12	22.49	.93	19:27	

N = 764

N = 2049

Continued on Next Page

TABLE 6-4. Continued

	Age 40–49				Age 50–59				
%	Balke Treadmill (time)	$\dot{V}O_{2\ Max}$ (ml/kg/min)	12 Min Run Distance (miles)	1.5 Mile Run (time)	Balke Treadmill (time)	$\dot{V}O_{2\ Max}$ (ml/kg/min)	12 Min Run Distance (miles)	1.5 Mile Run (time)	
99	22:00	46.75	1.61	10:47	18:44	42.04	1.48	12:28	
95	18:00	40.98	1.45	12:51	15:07	36.81	1.33	14:20	S
90	17:00	39.53	1.41	13:22	14:00	35.20	1.29	14:55	
85	15:35	37.49	1.35	14:06	12:53	33.59	1.24	15:29	E
80	14:45	36.28	1.32	14:31	12:00	32.31	1.21	15:57	
75	13:56	35.11	1.29	14:57	11:43	39.90	1.20	16:05	
70	13:00	33.76	1.25	15:16	11:00	30.87	1.17	16:27	
65	12:30	33.04	.23	15:41	10:14	29.76	1.14	16:51	
60	12:00	32.31	.21	15:57	10:00	29.43	1.13	16:58	G
55	11:30	31.59	.19	16:12	9:30	28.70	1.11	17:14	
50	11:00	30.87	.17	16:27	9:10	28.22	1.10	17:24	
45	10:48	30.58	1.16	16:34	9:00	27.98	1.09	17:29	F
40	10:01	29.45	1.13	16:58	8:13	26.85	1.06	17:55	
35	10:00	29.43	1.12	16:59	7:43	26.13	1.04	18:09	
30	9:11	28.25	1.10	17:24	7:16	25.48	1.02	18:23	
25	9:00	27.98	1.09	17:29	7:00	25.09	1.01	18:31	
20	8:00	26.54	1.05	18:00	6:25	24.25	.98	18:49	P
15	7:20	25.57	1.02	18:21	6:00	23.65	.97	19:02	
10	7:00	25.09	1.01	18:31	5:05	22.33	.93	19:30	
5	5:55	23.53	.96	19:05	4:14	21.10	.90	19:57	VP
1	4:00	20.76	.89	20:04	2:36	18.74	.83	20:47	

N = 1630   N = 878

Continued on Next Page

TABLE 6-4. Continued

		Age 60+			
%	Balke Treadmill (time)	$\dot{V}O_{2\ Max}$ (ml/kg/min)	12 Min Run Distance (miles)	1.5 Mile Run (time)	
99	20:25	44.47	1.55	11:36	
95	15:34	37.46	1.35	14:06	S
90	14:00	35.20	1.29	14:55	
85	12:00	32.31	1.21	15:57	
80	11:15	31.23	1.18	16:20	E
75	11:00	30.87	1.17	16:27	
70	10:00	29.43	1.13	16:58	
65	9:00	27.98	1.09	17:29	
60	8:28	27.21	1.07	17:46	G
55	8:00	26.54	1.05	18:00	
50	7:30	25.82	1.03	18:16	
45	7:00	25.09	1.01	18:31	
40	6:35	24.49	.99	18:44	F
35	6:16	24.03	.98	18:54	
30	6:08	23.80	.97	18:59	
25	6:00	23.65	.97	19:02	
20	5:24	22.78	.94	19:21	P
15	5:00	22.21	.93	19:33	
10	4:00	20.76	.89	20:04	
5	3:15	19.68	.86	20:23	VP
1	2:00	17.87	.81	21:06	

N = 202

*Data provided by the Institute for Aerobics Research, Dallas, TX (1994). S, superior; E, excellent; G, good; F, fair; P, poor; VP, very poor.

118

TABLE 6–5. LEG STRENGTH (MEN)*

1 REPETITION MAXIMUM LEG PRESS

LEG PRESS WEIGHT RATIO = $\dfrac{\text{WEIGHT PUSHED}}{\text{BODY WEIGHT}}$

%	\<20	20–29	30–39	40–49	50–59	60+	
99	>2.82	>2.40	>2.20	>2.02	>1.90	>1.80	
95	2.82	2.40	2.20	2.02	1.90	1.80	S
90	2.53	2.27	2.07	1.92	1.80	1.73	
85	2.40	2.18	1.99	1.86	1.75	1.68	
80	2.28	2.13	1.93	1.82	1.71	1.62	E
75	2.18	2.09	1.89	1.78	1.68	1.58	
70	2.15	2.05	1.85	1.74	1.64	1.56	
65	2.10	2.01	1.81	1.71	1.61	1.52	
60	2.04	1.97	1.77	1.68	1.58	1.49	G
55	2.01	1.94	1.74	1.65	1.55	1.46	
50	1.95	1.91	1.71	1.62	1.52	1.43	
45	1.93	1.87	1.68	1.59	1.50	1.40	
40	1.90	1.83	1.65	1.57	1.46	1.38	F
35	1.89	1.78	1.62	1.54	1.42	1.34	
30	1.82	1.74	1.59	1.51	1.39	1.30	
25	1.80	1.68	1.56	1.48	1.36	1.27	
20	1.70	1.63	1.52	1.44	1.32	1.25	P
15	1.61	1.58	1.48	1.40	1.28	1.21	
10	1.57	1.51	1.43	1.35	1.22	1.16	
5	1.46	1.42	1.34	1.27	1.15	1.08	VP
1	\<1.46	\<1.42	\<1.34	\<1.27	\<1.15	\<1.08	
N =	60	424	1909	2089	1286	347	

TOTAL N = 6115

*Data provided by the Institute for Aerobics Research, Dallas, TX (1994). S, superior; E, excellent; G, good; F, fair; P, poor; VP, very poor.

exercise-induced ST-segment changes, but normal angiograms, were followed for seven years, there was no increased incidence of cardiac events compared with subjects who had no ST-segment changes.[2] In another study,[3] GXT data were used to examine cardiac events (infarction or death) in 3,617 asymptomatic, hypercholesterolemic

TABLE 6–6. LEG STRENGTH (WOMEN)*

1 REPETITION MAXIMUM LEG PRESS

LEG PRESS WEIGHT RATIO = WEIGHT PUSHED / BODY WEIGHT

	Age						
%	<20	20–29	30–39	40–49	50–59	60+	
99	>1.88	>1.98	>1.68	>1.57	>1.43	>1.43	
95	1.88	1.98	1.68	1.57	1.43	1.43	S
90	1.85	1.82	1.61	1.48	1.37	1.32	
85	1.81	1.76	1.52	1.40	1.31	1.32	
80	1.71	1.68	1.47	1.37	1.25	1.18	E
75	1.69	1.65	1.42	1.33	1.20	1.16	
70	1.65	1.58	1.39	1.29	1.17	1.13	
65	1.62	1.53	1.36	1.27	1.12	1.08	
60	1.59	1.50	1.33	1.23	1.10	1.04	G
55	1.51	1.47	1.31	1.20	1.08	1.01	
50	1.45	1.44	1.27	1.18	1.05	.99	
45	1.42	1.40	1.24	1.15	1.02	.97	
40	1.38	1.37	1.21	1.13	.99	.93	F
35	1.33	1.32	1.18	1.11	.97	.90	
30	1.29	1.27	1.15	1.08	.95	.88	
25	1.25	1.26	1.12	1.06	.92	.86	
20	1.22	1.22	1.09	1.02	.88	.85	P
15	1.19	1.18	1.05	.97	.84	.80	
10	1.09	1.14	1.00	.94	.78	.72	
5	1.06	.99	.96	.85	.72	.63	VP
1	<1.06	<.99	<.96	<.85	<.72	<.63	
N =	20	192	281	337	192	44	
TOTAL N = 1166							

*Data provided by the Institute for Aerobics Research, Dallas, TX (1994). S, superior; E, excellent; G, good; F, fair; P, poor; VP, very poor.

men. Exercise testing only identified one-third of the men who had cardiac events, and 95% of abnormal responders were false positives. Such results in a population initially screened for risk factors (which increases pre-test prevalence of disease) strongly urges against the use of exercise testing as a screening tool for CAD in apparently healthy

TABLE 6–7. UPPER BODY STRENGTH (MEN)*

1 REPETITION MAXIMUM BENCH PRESS

BENCH PRESS WEIGHT RATIO = WEIGHT PUSHED / BODY WEIGHT

%	<20	20–29	30–39	40–49	50–59	60+	
99	>1.76	>1.63	>1.35	>1.20	>1.05	>.94	
95	1.76	1.63	1.35	1.20	1.05	.94	S
90	1.46	1.48	1.24	1.10	.97	.89	
85	1.38	1.37	1.17	1.04	.93	.84	
80	1.34	1.32	1.12	1.00	.90	.82	E
75	1.29	1.26	1.08	.96	.87	.79	
70	1.24	1.22	1.04	.93	.84	.77	
65	1.23	1.18	1.01	.90	.81	.74	
60	1.19	1.14	.98	.88	.79	.72	G
55	1.16	1.10	.96	.86	.77	.70	
50	1.13	1.06	.93	.84	.75	.68	
45	1.10	1.03	.90	.82	.73	.67	
40	1.06	.99	.88	.80	.71	.66	F
35	1.01	.96	.86	.78	.70	.65	
30	.96	.93	.83	.76	.68	.63	
25	.93	.90	.81	.74	.66	.60	
20	.89	.88	.78	.72	.63	.57	P
15	.86	.84	.75	.69	.60	.56	
10	.81	.80	.71	.65	.57	.53	
5	.76	.72	.65	.59	.53	.49	VP
1	<.76	<.72	<.65	<.59	<.53	<.49	
N =	60	425	1909	2090	1279	343	

TOTAL N = 6106

*Data provided by the Institute for Aerobics Research, Dallas, TX (1994). S, superior; E, excellent; G, good; F, fair; P, poor; VP, very poor.

adults. Such a use for GXT is ineffective and has the potential to cause harm (psychological, work and insurance status, costs for more tests, etc.) by misclassifying a large percentage of those without CAD as having disease.

Given current approaches, it is best to screen only those who request it, those with multiple risk factors, and those

TABLE 6–8. UPPER BODY STRENGTH (WOMEN)*

1 REPETITION MAXIMUM BENCH PRESS

BENCH PRESS WEIGHT RATIO = WEIGHT PUSHED / BODY WEIGHT

%	<20	20–29	30–39	40–49	50–59	60+	
99	>.88	>1.01	>.82	>.77	>.68	>.72	
95	.88	1.01	.82	.77	.68	.72	S
90	.83	.90	.76	.71	.61	.64	
85	.81	.83	.72	.66	.57	.59	
80	.77	.80	.70	.62	.55	.54	E
75	.76	.77	.65	.60	.53	.53	
70	.74	.74	.63	.57	.52	.51	
65	.70	.72	.62	.55	.50	.48	
60	.65	.70	.60	.54	.48	.47	G
55	.64	.68	.58	.53	.47	.46	
50	.63	.65	.57	.52	.46	.45	
45	.60	.63	.55	.51	.45	.44	
40	.58	.59	.53	.50	.44	.43	F
35	.57	.58	.52	.48	.43	.41	
30	.56	.56	.51	.47	.42	.40	
25	.55	.53	.49	.45	.41	.39	
20	.53	.51	.47	.43	.39	.38	P
15	.52	.50	.45	.42	.38	.36	
10	.50	.480	.42	.38	.37	.33	
5	.41	.436	.39	.35	.305	.26	VP
1	<.41	<.436	<.39	<.35	<.305	<.26	
N =	20	191	379	333	189	42	

TOTAL N = 1154

*Data provided by the Institute for Aerobics Research, Dallas, TX (1994). S, superior; E, excellent; G, good; F, fair; P, poor; VP, very poor.

with worrisome medical histories or a strong family history of premature cardiovascular disease. It is likewise difficult to choose a chronological age beyond which exercise testing becomes valuable as a screening tool prior to beginning an exercise program, since physiologi-

TABLE 6–9. PUSH-UP NORMS (MEN)*

%	Age					
	20–29	30–39	40–49	50–59	60+	
99	100	86	64	51	39	
95	62	52	40	39	28	S
90	57	46	36	30	26	
85	51	41	34	28	24	
80	47	39	30	25	23	E
75	44	36	29	24	22	
70	41	34	26	21	21	
65	39	31	25	20	20	
60	37	30	24	19	18	G
55	35	29	22	17	16	
50	33	27	21	15	15	
45	31	25	19	14	12	
40	29	24	18	13	10	F
35	27	21	16	11	9	
30	26	20	15	10	8	
25	24	19	13	9.5	7	
20	22	17	11	9	6	P
15	19	15	10	7	5	
10	18	13	9	6	4	
5	13	9	5	3	2	VP
N =	1045	790	364	172	26	

TOTAL N = 2397

*Data provided by the Institute for Aerobics Research, Dallas, TX (1994). S, superior; E, excellent; G, good; F, fair; P, poor; VP, very poor.

cal age often differs from chronological age. In general, if the exercise is more strenuous than vigorous walking, the guidelines in Table 2–7 are recommended. The potential problems resulting from mass screening must be considered and the results of such testing must be applied using the predictive model and Bayesian statistics. Test results should be considered as probability statements and not as absolutes.

TABLE 6–10. MODIFIED PUSH-UP NORMS (WOMEN)*

%	Age					
	20–29	30–39	40–49	50–59	60+	
99	70	56	60	31	20	
95	45	39	33	28	20	S
90	42	36	28	25	17	
85	39	33	26	23	15	
80	36	31	24	21	15	E
75	34	29	21	20	15	
70	32	28	20	19	14	
65	31	26	19	18	13	
60	30	24	18	17	12	G
55	29	23	17	15	12	
50	26	21	15	13	8	
45	25	20	14	13	6	
40	23	19	13	12	5	F
35	22	17	11	10	4	
30	20	15	10	9	3	
25	19	14	9	8	2	
20	17	11	6	6	2	P
15	15	9	4	4	1	
10	12	8	2	1	0	
5	9	4	1	0	0	VP
N =	579	411	246	105	12	
TOTAL N = 1353						

*Data provided by the Institute for Aerobics Research, Dallas, TX (1994).
S, superior; E, excellent; G, good; F, fair; P, poor; VP, very poor.

INTERPRETATION OF RESPONSES TO GRADED EXERCISE TESTING

EXERCISE CAPACITY

Estimated or measured maximal exercise intensity provides important information about cardiovascular fitness and prognosis. Population specific nomograms (Fig. 5–1) may be used when appropriate to compare the peak METs

TABLE 6–11. MUSCULAR ENDURANCE (MEN)*

1 MINUTE SIT-UP: NUMBER

%	<20	20–29	30–39	40–49	50–59	60+	
99	>62	>55	>51	>47	>43	>39	
95	62	55	51	47	43	39	S
90	55	52	48	43	39	35	
85	53	49	45	40	36	31	
80	51	47	43	39	35	30	E
75	50	46	42	37	33	28	
70	48	45	41	36	31	26	
65	48	44	40	35	30	24	
60	47	42	39	34	28	22	G
55	46	41	37	32	27	21	
50	45	40	36	31	26	20	
45	42	39	36	30	25	19	
40	41	38	35	29	24	19	F
35	39	37	33	28	22	18	
30	38	35	32	27	21	17	
25	37	35	31	26	20	16	
20	36	33	30	24	19	15	P
15	34	32	28	22	17	13	
10	33	30	26	20	15	10	
5	27	27	23	17	12	7	VP
1	<27	<27	<23	<17	<12	<7	
N =	46	312	1431	1558	919	205	

TOTAL N = 4471

*Data provided by the Institute for Aerobics Research, Dallas, TX (1994). S, superior; E, excellent; G, good; F, fair; P, poor; VP, very poor.

achieved on a GXT with the expected maximal intensity for a given age and activity status. Exercise capacity is not strongly related to ventricular function, and abnormal ventricular function does not always result in low exercise capacity. Various objective and subjective indicators are useful to confirm that a maximal effort has been performed during graded exercise testing:

TABLE 6-12. MUSCULAR ENDURANCE (WOMEN)*

1 MINUTE SIT-UP: NUMBER

%	<20	20–29	30–39	40–49	50–59	60+	
			Age				
99	>55	>51	>42	>38	>30	>28	
95	55	51	42	38	30	28	S
90	54	49	40	34	29	26	
85	49	45	38	32	25	20	
80	46	44	35	29	24	17	E
75	40	42	33	28	22	15	
70	38	41	32	27	22	12	
65	37	39	30	25	21	12	
60	36	38	29	24	20	11	G
55	35	37	28	23	19	10	
50	34	35	27	22	17	8	
45	34	34	26	21	16	8	
40	32	32	25	20	14	6	F
35	30	31	24	19	12	5	
30	29	30	22	17	12	4	
25	29	28	21	16	11	4	
20	28	27	20	14	10	3	P
15	27	24	18	13	7	2	
10	25	23	15	10	6	1	
5	25	18	11	7	5	0	VP
1	<25	<18	<11	<7	<5	<0	
N =	15	144	289	249	137	26	

TOTAL N = 860

*Data provided by the Institute for Aerobics Research, Dallas, TX (1994).
S, superior; E, excellent; G, good; F, fair; P, poor; VP, very poor.

- Failure of HR to increase with further increases in intensity
- A plateau in oxygen uptake (or failure to increase oxygen uptake by 150 ml/minute) with increased workload.[4] While this is the criterion measure, a plateau is infrequently seen during continuous graded exercise tests
- R >1.15
- A venous lactic acid concentration of >8 mmol has also been used; however, this requires a mixed venous blood sample and there is great interindividual variability in this response
- RPE >17 (6–20 scale)

TABLE 6–13. FLEXIBILITY (MEN)*

SIT AND REACH: INCHES

%	<20	29–29	30–39	40–49	50–59	60+	
			Age				
99	>23.4	>23.0	>22.0	>21.3	>20.5	>20.0	
95	23.4	23.0	22.0	21.3	20.5	20.0	S
90	22.6	21.8	21.0	20.0	19.0	19.0	
85	22.4	21.0	20.0	19.3	18.3	18.0	
80	21.7	20.5	19.5	18.5	17.5	17.3	E
75	21.4	20.0	19.0	18.0	17.0	16.5	
70	20.7	19.5	18.5	17.5	16.5	15.5	
65	19.8	19.0	18.0	17.0	16.0	15.0	
60	19.0	18.5	17.5	16.3	15.5	14.5	G
55	18.7	18.0	17.0	16.0	15.0	14.0	
50	18.0	17.5	16.5	15.3	14.5	13.5	
45	17.3	17.0	16.0	15.0	14.0	13.0	
40	16.5	16.5	15.5	14.3	13.3	12.5	F
35	16.0	16.0	15.0	14.0	12.5	12.0	
30	15.5	15.5	14.5	13.3	12.0	11.3	
25	14.1	15.0	13.8	12.5	11.2	10.5	
20	13.2	14.4	13.0	12.0	10.5	10.0	P
15	11.9	13.5	12.0	11.0	9.7	9.0	
10	10.5	12.3	11.0	10.0	8.5	8.0	
5	9.4	10.5	9.3	8.3	7.0	5.8	VP
1	<9.4	<10.5	<9.3	<8.3	<7.0	<5.8	
N =	56	422	1,906	2,090	1,278	344	

TOTAL N = 6096

*Data provided by the Institute for Aerobics Research, Dallas, TX (1994).
S, superior; E, excellent; G, good; F, fair; P, poor; VP, very poor

TABLE 6–14. FLEXIBILITY (WOMEN)*

SIT AND REACH: INCHES

%	<20	20–29	30–39	40–49	50–59	60+	
			Age				
99	>24.3	>24.0	>24.0	>22.8	>23.0	>23.0	
95	24.3	24.5	24.0	22.8	23.0	23.0	S
90	24.3	23.8	22.5	21.5	21.5	21.8	
85	22.5	23.0	22.0	21.3	21.0	19.5	
80	22.5	22.5	21.5	20.5	20.3	19.0	E
75	22.3	22.0	21.0	20.0	20.0	18.0	
70	22.0	21.5	20.5	19.8	19.3	17.5	
65	21.8	21.0	20.3	19.1	19.0	17.5	
60	21.5	20.5	20.0	19.0	18.5	17.0	G
55	21.3	20.3	19.5	18.5	18.0	17.0	
50	21.0	20.0	19.0	18.0	17.9	16.4	
45	20.5	19.5	18.5	18.0	17.0	16.1	
40	20.5	19.3	18.3	17.3	16.8	15.5	F
35	20.0	19.0	17.8	17.0	16.0	15.2	
30	19.5	18.3	17.3	16.5	15.5	14.4	
25	19.0	17.8	16.8	16.0	15.3	13.6	
20	18.5	17.0	16.5	15.0	14.8	13.0	P
15	17.8	16.4	15.5	14.0	14.0	11.5	
10	14.5	15.4	14.4	13.0	13.0	11.5	
5	14.5	14.1	12.0	10.5	12.3	9.2	VP
1	<14.5	<14.1	<12.0	<10.5	<12.3	<9.2	
N =	19	183	376	332	192	44	

TOTAL N = 1146

*Data provided by the Institute for Aerobics Research, Dallas, TX (1994).
S, superior; E, excellent; G, good; F, fair; P, poor; VP, very poor.

Achievement of age-predicted maximal heart rate (HR_{max}) should not be used as an absolute test end-point, nor as an indication that effort has been maximal, due to its high intersubject variability (see following).

HEART RATE RESPONSE

HR_{max} may be predicted from age using any of several published equations (see Appendix D). The relationship between age and HR_{max} for a large sample of subjects (i.e., the regression equation) is reproducible; however, interindividual variability is high (standard deviation = 10–15 beats/min). As a result, there is potential for considerable error in the use of methods that extrapolate submaximal test data to an age-predicted HR_{max}. Figure 6–1[5] presents observed HR_{max} responses to graded exercise versus age, based on different exercise test modalities and in different subject categories. $\dot{V}O_{2max}$, anthropometric measures such as height and weight, and body composition do not independently influence HR_{max}.

Figure 6–2[6] presents the HR and BP responses of more than 700 men to maximal treadmill exercise and provides percentile responses for comparative purposes.

BLOOD PRESSURE RESPONSE

The normal blood pressure response to dynamic upright exercise consists of a progressive increase in systolic pressure (SBP), no change or a slight decrease in diastolic pressure (DBP), and a widening of the pulse pressure. The following are key points concerning interpretation of the blood pressure response to progressive dynamic exercise:

- A drop in SBP, or failure of SBP to increase, with increased exercise intensity should be viewed as an abnormal test response. Exercise-induced decreases in SBP (exercise-induced hypotension, EIH) may occur in patients with CAD, valvular heart disease, cardiomyopathies, and various arrhythmias. Occasionally, patients without clinically significant heart disease will exhibit EIH due to anti-hypertensive therapy, prolonged strenuous exercise, and vasovagal responses. Although the prognosis of EIH has not been examined in post-MI patients, an abnormal SBP response to exercise is associated with subsequent cardiac events in this population and is corrected by CABG[7]

- The normal post-exercise response is a progressive decline in SBP. During passive recovery in an upright posture, SBP may decrease abruptly due to peripheral pooling (and usually normalizes upon resuming the supine position). SBP may remain below pre-test resting values for several hours after the test. DBP may also drop during the post-exercise period
- Double product (SBP × HR) is an indicator of myocardial oxygen demand. Signs and symptoms of ischemia often occur at a reproducible double product
- While an increase in DBP with increasing exercise intensity can be associated with CAD, it is better viewed as an indicator of labile hypertension
- In patients on vasodilators, calcium channel blockers, ACE inhibitors, and α- and β-blockers, the BP response to exercise is variably attenuated, and cannot be accurately predicted in the absence of clinical test data

The normative data shown in Figure 6–2 were based on an exclusively male sample. Mean peak SBP and DBP by age and gender are provided in Table 6–15.[8]

INTERPRETATION OF CLINICAL TEST DATA

Prior to interpreting clinical test data, it is important to consider the purpose of the test (e.g., diagnostic or prognostic) and patient conditions that may have an effect on the GXT or its interpretation. Medical conditions influencing test interpretation include orthopedic disabilities, pulmonary disease, obesity, neurological disorders, and significant deconditioning. Medication effects (see Appendix A) and resting ECG abnormalities must also be considered, especially resting ST-segment

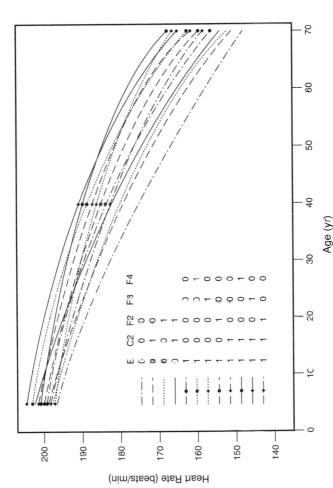

FIG. 6–1. Plots from literature review of studies involving multiple different types of dynamic exercise. Under *E* (ergometer), *C* = bicycle, and *1* = treadmill; under *C2* (European), *F2* (sedentary), *F3* (active), and *F4* (endurance trained), *1* = class inclusion (that is, a member of that category), and *0* = class exclusion. Reprinted with permission from Reference 5.

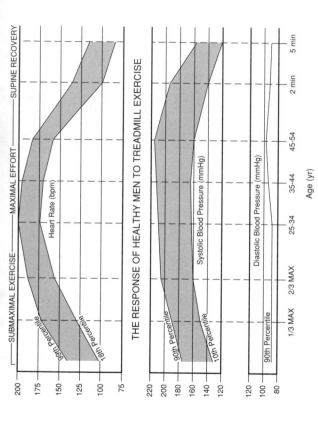

FIG. 6–2. The hemodynamic responses of over 700 healthy men to maximal treadmill exercise. *Bands* represent 80% of the population, with 10% having values exceeding the upper limit and 10% having lower values. Reprinted with permission from Reference 6.

TABLE 6–15. MEAN (±S.D.) PEAK SBP AND DBP (mm HG)
DURING MAXIMAL TREADMILL EXERCISE*

Age	Men		Women	
	SBP	DBP	SBP	DBP
18–29	182±22	69±13	155±19	67±12
30–39	182±20	76±12	158±20	72±12
40–49	186±22	78±12	165±22	76±12
50–59	192±22	82±12	175±23	78±11
60–69	195±23	83±12	181±23	79±11
70–79	191±27	81±13	196±23	83±11

Reprinted with permission from Reference 8.

changes secondary to conduction defects, LVH, and other conditions.

While whole body oxygen consumption ($\dot{V}O_2$) and myocardial oxygen consumption ($m\dot{V}O_2$) are directly related, that relationship can be altered by training, drugs, and disease. For example, exercise-induced ischemia may cause cardiac dysfunction, exercise impairment, and an abnormal SBP response. While the severity of ischemia (or the amount of myocardium in jeopardy) is inversely related to the exercise intensity achieved, ejection fraction does not correlate well with $\dot{V}O_{2max}$.[6,9] Silent ischemia does not appear to affect exercise capacity in CAD patients.[10]

ECG WAVEFORMS

Appendix C provides information to aid in the interpretation of the resting and exercise electrocardiograms. Additional information is provided here with respect to specific interpretation of exercise-induced changes in ECG variables. The normal ECG response to exercise includes:

- Minor and insignificant changes in P wave morphology
- Superimposition of the P and T waves of successive beats
- Increases in septal Q wave amplitude
- Slight decreases in R wave amplitude
- Increases in T wave amplitude (although wide variability exists among subjects)
- Minimal shortening of the QRS duration
- Depression of the j-point
- Rate-related shortening of the QT interval

On the other hand, some changes in ECG wave morphology may be indicative of underlying pathology. For example, while QRS duration tends to decrease slightly with exercise (and increasing HR) in normal subjects, it may increase in patients with either angina or LV dysfunction.

Exercise-induced P wave changes corresponding to P-pulmonale or P-mitrale are rarely seen and of questionable significance. Many factors affect R-wave amplitude, and R-wave amplitude changes during exercise have no independent predictive power.[12]

ST SEGMENT CHANGES

ST segment changes are widely accepted criteria for myocardial ischemia and injury. Interpretation of ST segments may be affected by the resting ECG configuration (bundle branch blocks, left ventricular hypertrophy, etc.) and pharmacological agents (e.g., digitalis preparations). There may be j-point depression and tall peaked T-waves at high exercise intensities and during recovery in normal subjects. Depression of the j-point leads to marked ST-segment upsloping and results from competition between normal repolarization and delayed terminal depolarization forces, rather than ischemia.[13] On the other hand, exercise-induced myocardial ischemia can manifest itself by three different types of ST-segment changes on the ECG:

ST-segment elevation
- ST-segment elevation (early repolarization) may be seen in the normal resting ECG. Increasing HR may cause normally elevated ST-segments to return to the isoelectric line
- ST-segment elevation indicates myocardial injury (i.e. an acute or evolving infarct) when present in conjunction with significant Q-waves
- Chronic resting ST-segment elevation in conjunction with significant Q waves may be indicative of wall motion abnormalities, including aneurysm
- Exercise-induced ST-elevation on an otherwise normal ECG (except in aVR or V_{1-2}) represents transmural ischemia, is very arrhythmogenic, and localizes the ischemia[14]

ST-segment normalization or absence of change
- One manifestation of ischemia can be normalization of resting ST-segments. ECG abnormalities at rest, including T-wave inversion and ST-segment depression, may return to normal during attacks of angina and during exercise in some CAD patients. This normalization of ST-segment depression should be treated as ST-segment elevation[15]

ST-segment depression
- ST-segment depression (depression of the j-point and the slope over the following 60 msec) is the most common manifestation of exercise-induced myocardial ischemia
- Horizontal or downward sloping ST-segment depression is more indicative of subendocardial ischemia than upsloping depression
- Slowly upsloping ST-segment depression should be considered a borderline response, and added emphasis should be placed on other clinical and exercise variables

- ST-depression does not localize the area of ischemia nor indicate which coronary artery is involved
- The more leads with (apparent) ischemic ST-segment shifts, the more severe the disease
- Significant ST-depression occurring only in recovery is not likely to represent a false-positive response[16]

Examples of the various criteria for ischemic ST-segment displacement, as well as some waveform changes previously discussed, are shown in Figure 6–3.

A gradual decrease in T-wave amplitude is usually observed in all leads during early exercise. At maximal exercise the T-wave amplitude begins to increase, and at one-minute recovery the amplitude is equivalent to resting values, except in leads II, aVF and V_2, where the T-wave amplitude is usually greater than at rest.

In patients with left bundle branch block (LBBB), the ST-segment response to exercise testing cannot be used to diagnose ischemia.[17] In rate dependent LBBB, the HR at onset may be helpful in diagnosing CAD.[18] In right bundle branch block (RBBB), exercise-induced ST-segment displacement in the anterior precordial leads (V_1,V_2, and V_3) should not be used to diagnose ischemia; however, ST-segment changes in the lateral leads (V_4, V_5, and V_6) may be indicative of ischemia even in the presence of RBBB.[19]

ARRHYTHMIAS

Exercise-associated arrhythmias occur in healthy subjects as well as patients with cardiac disease. Increased sympathetic drive and changes in extracellular and intracellular electrolytes, pH, and oxygen tension contribute to disturbances in myocardial and conducting tissue automaticity and re-entry, which are major mechanisms of arrhythmias.

Supraventricular Arrhythmias. Isolated premature atrial contractions (PACs) are common and require no special precautions. Chaotic atrial rhythm, atrial flutter, or atrial fibrillation may occur in organic heart disease or may reflect endocrine, metabolic, or drug effects (hyperthyroidism, alcoholic cardiomyopathy, alcohol consumption, and digoxin toxicity).

Sustained supraventricular tachycardia (SVT) is occasionally induced by exercise and may require pharmacological treatment or electroconversion if discontinuation of exercise or use of vagal reflex maneuvers fail to abolish the rhythm. Patients who experience exercise-induced SVT may be evaluated by repeating the GXT after appropriate treatment.

Ventricular Arrhythmias. Isolated premature ventricular complexes or contractions (PVCs) occur during exercise in 30 to 40% of healthy subjects and in 50 to 60% of patients with CAD. In some individuals, graded exercise induces PVCs while in others it reduces their occurrence. The significance of induction or suppression of PVCs during exercise testing has not been fully determined. Significant CAD may be found in patients who show rate suppression of PVCs during exercise, however. The daily variability of PVC activity is considerable.

PVCs are usually only ominous when occurring in patients with a history of sudden death, cardiomyopathy, valvular heart disease, or severe ischemia.[20] Nonsustained exercise-induced ventricular tachycardia during routine treadmill testing is not associated with other complications during testing or with increased cardiovascular mortality.[21] The prevalence of exercise-induced ventricular tachycardia is low in most clinical laboratories and usually consists of only three consecutive beats.

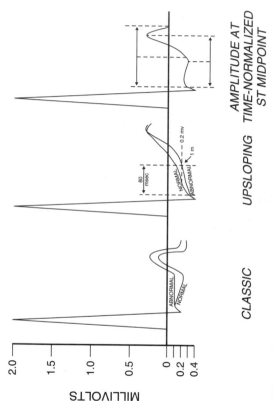

MILLIVOLTS

CLASSIC   UPSLOPING   AMPLITUDE AT TIME-NORMALIZED ST MIDPOINT

FIG. 6–3. Standard visual and computer criteria for identifying ischemia. As shown, there are different ways of calculating the measurements. Blomqvist recommended using the end of the T wave for measuring the midpoint of the ST segment, but Simoons used the peak of the T wave. This change was made to have a more stable end point, since the end of the T wave is much more difficult to find

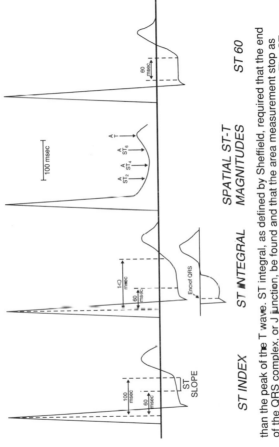

ST INDEX   ST INTEGRAL   SPATIAL ST-T
MAGNITUDES   ST 60

than the peak of the T wave. ST integral, as defined by Sheffield, required that the end of the QRS complex, or J junction, be found and that the area measurement stop as soon as the ST segment crossed the isoelectric line or as the T wave began. The ST integral used by most commercial systems initiates the area at a fixed period after the R wave and then encs 80 msec thereafter.

Criteria for terminating exercise tests based on ventricular ectopy include: increasing frequency of PVCs, multiform appearance, and coupling and salvos of ventricular tachycardia. The decision to terminate a GXT may also be influenced by simultaneous evidence of ischemia or symptoms (see Table 5–4).

PREDICTIVE VALUE OF EXERCISE TESTING

The predictive value of ECG exercise testing for the detection of CAD is controlled by the principles of conditional probability (Table 6–16). The factors that determine the predictive outcome of exercise testing (and other diagnostic tests) are the *sensitivity* and *specificity* of the test procedure and the *prevalence* of the disease or condition in the population tested. Sensitivity and specificity deter-

---

TABLE 6–16. SENSITIVITY, SPECIFICITY, AND PREDICTIVE VALUE OF DIAGNOSTIC GRADED EXERCISE TESTING

Sensitivity = TP/(TP + FN) =
  the percentage of patients with CAD who will have an abnormal test
Specificity = TN/(TN + FP) =
  the percentage of patients without CAD who will have a negative test
Predictive Value (positive test) = TP/(TP + FP) =
  the percentage of patients with a positive test result who have CAD
Predictive Value (negative test) = TN/(TN + FN) =
  the percentage of patients with a negative test who do not have CAD

Key: TP = True Positive (+Exercise Test and CAD); FP = False Positive (+Exercise Test and no CAD); TN = True Negative (–Exercise Test and no CAD); FN = False Negative (–Exercise Test and CAD).

mine how effective the test is in making correct diagnoses in diseased and nondiseased individuals, respectively. Disease prevalence is an important determinant of the *predictive value* of the test.

SENSITIVITY

Sensitivity refers to the percent of patients tested who have CAD and who show positive (abnormal) test results. Exercise ECG sensitivity for the detection of CAD is usually based on subsequent angiographically determined coronary artery stenosis of 50 to 70% in at least 1 vessel. A true positive GXT (based on ST-segment depression of ≥ 1.0 mm) correctly identifies a patient with CAD. False negative test results show no or nondiagnostic ECG changes and fail to identify patients with true CAD. Therefore, the sensitivity of ECG exercise testing is reduced, depending on the number of false negative tests.

Common factors that contribute to false negative results of exercise tests are summarized in Table 6–17. Test sensitivity is decreased by inadequate stress, insufficient ECG lead monitoring, and drugs that alter cardiac work responses to exercise or reduce ischemia (beta blockers,

TABLE 6–17. CAUSES OF FALSE NEGATIVE TEST RESULTS

1. Failure to reach an ischemic threshold
2. Monitoring an insufficent number of leads to detect ECG changes
3. Failure to recognize non-ECG signs and symptoms that may be associated with underlying disease, e.g., hypotension
4. Angiographically significant disease compensated by collateral circulation
5. Musculoskeletal limitations to exercise preceding cardiac abnormalities
6. Technical or observer error

nitrates, and calcium channel blocking agents). Pre-existing ECG changes, such as LBBB, limit the ability to interpret ST-segment changes as ischemic ECG responses. If the criteria for a positive test are increased (e.g., from 1.0 to 2.0 mm ST depression), overall sensitivity decreases because a significant number of true positive tests (those with between 1.0 and 2.0 mm of ST-segment depression) are excluded.

SPECIFICITY

The specificity of exercise tests refers to the percent of normal subjects (without CAD) who show a negative or non-diagnostic stress test. A true negative test correctly identifies a person without disease. Specificity is reduced by false positive tests in persons without CAD. Many conditions may cause individuals to have false positive exercise ECG responses (Table 6–18).

Hyperventilation alters repolarization and thus causes nonischemic ST-segment changes in some people. Hyperventilation should be performed post-exercise on select

TABLE 6–18. CAUSES OF FALSE POSITIVE TEST RESULTS

1. Resting repolarization abnormalities (e.g., LBBB)
2. Cardiac hypertrophy
3. Accelerated conduction defects (e.g., W-P-W syndrome)
4. Digitalis
5. Nonischemic cardiomyopathy
6. Hypokalemia
7. Vasoregulatory abnormalities
8. Mitral valve prolapse
9. Pericardial disorders
10. Technical or observer error
11. Coronary spasm in the absence of significant CAD
12. Anemia
13. Female gender

patients who have an abnormal response rather than being routinely performed, as such changes are unusual and have rarely been responsible for false-positive tests. Hypertension does not increase the likelihood of a false-positive test.

Reported values for the specificity and sensitivity of exercise ECG responses vary substantially. The exercise test has a higher sensitivity in individuals with triple vessel disease than in those with single vessel disease. The variation has been attributed to significant differences in patient selection, test protocols, ECG criteria for a positive test, and angiographic definition of CAD. In studies that controlled these factors, the pooled results show a sensitivity of 68% and a specificity of 79%.[22]

PREDICTIVE VALUE

The predictive value of exercise testing is a measure of how accurately a test result (positive or negative) correctly identifies the presence or absence of CAD in patients tested. That is, the predictive value of an abnormal test is the percentage of those persons with an abnormal test who have the disease. Predictive value cannot be directly estimated from a test's demonstrated specificity or sensitivity. Predictive value is dependent upon the prevalence of disease in the population tested. Examples of this are shown in Table 6–19.

Non-ECG criteria, such as duration of exercise or maximal MET level, SBP response, HR_{max}, rate-pressure product, and symptoms of angina or dyspnea, must be considered in the overall interpretation of exercise test results. Multivariate analysis of these variables in combination with ECG criteria show improved overall sensitivity for detection of CAD and higher specificity for the absence of multivessel CAD in patients with probable angina.

TABLE 6–19. TEST PERFORMANCE VS. PREDICTIVE VALUE AND RISK RATIO: A MODEL IN A POPULATION OF 10,000

Disease Prevalence	Subjects	Number with Abnormal Test Results	Test Performance	Number with Normal Test Results
5%	500 diseased	450 (TP)	90% sensitivity	50 (FN)
		350 (TP)	70% sensitivity	150 (FN)
	9500 nondiseased	2850 (FP)	70% specificity	6650 (TN)
		950 (FP)	90% specificity	8550 (TN)
50%	5000 diseased	4500 (TP)	90% sensitivity	500 (FN)
		3500 (TP)	70% sensitivity	1500 (FN)
	5000 nondiseased	1500 (FP)	70% specificity	3500 (TN)
		500 (FP)	90% specificity	4500 (TN)

	Predictive Value of Abnormal Test		Risk ratio*	
Disease Prevalence	5	50	5	50
Sensitivity/Specificity				
70%/90%	27%	88%	27	3
90%/70%	14%	75%	14	5
90%/90%	32%	90%	64	9
66%/84%	18%	80%	9	3

*Times that for normal subjects.
Key: TP = true positive test result; FP = false positive test result; FN = false negative test result; TN = true negative test result.

COMPARISON WITH RADIONUCLIDE IMAGING

Radionuclide techniques are especially helpful in the evaluation of typical or atypical angina with apparent normal exercise or equivocal (discordant) ECGs and for the evaluation of probable false positive exercise ECG responses. In these cases, a rational incremental testing strategy for determining prognostic risk of CAD consists of clinical risk evaluation, evaluation of exercise-induced ST-segment depression, and radionuclide perfusion scintigraphy.

Numerous studies have demonstrated that thallium exercise testing is the usual second-level test in clarifying an abnormal ST-segment response in asymptomatic individuals. Those with positive ECG and thallium scan have a 2.6-fold relative risk for subsequent coronary events, independent of conventional risk factors.[23]

PROGNOSTIC APPLICATIONS OF THE EXERCISE TEST

Available literature supports the use of graded exercise testing as the first noninvasive step after the history, physical examination, and resting ECG in the prognostic evaluation of CAD patients. It accomplishes both of the purposes of prognostic testing: to provide information regarding the patient's status and to help make recommendations for optimal management. The exercise test results assist in decisions for selection of patients who should undergo coronary angiography. Simple clinical and exercise test scores can be used to decide which patients need interventions in order to improve their prognosis; these scores frequently obviate the need for cardiac catheterization. The VA score[24] has been validated for the male veteran population and the Duke score[25] (see Chapter 5) for the general population, including women.

The maximum amount of horizontal or downsloping ST-segment depression in exercise or recovery has been shown to be a powerful predictor of disease severity, with 2 mm ST-segment depression yielding a sensitivity of 55% and a specificity of 80% for prediction of severe angiographic disease.[26]

INTERPRETATION OF EXERCISE TESTS IN PULMONARY PATIENTS

The major abnormalities of cardiopulmonary exercise responses are ventilatory limitation and/or oxygen desaturation in patients with moderate to severe lung disease (asthma, COPD, and interstitial lung disease):

Ventilatory limitation
- Is assessed by calculating the $\dot{V}_E$max/MVV ratio (~50–70% in normal healthy individuals)
- A ratio of >70% (i.e., a low breathing reserve, BR) is indicative of ventilatory limitations

O_2 desaturation
- Gas exchange may be impaired during exercise in some patients with respiratory disease
- A decrease in S_aO_2 of at least 3% is necessary to indicate "significant" O_2 desaturation
- The resting (baseline) S_aO_2 and its position on the oxyhemoglobin curve is also important (e.g., a decrease in S_aO_2 from 91% at rest to 87% during exercise may lead to pulmonary vasoconstriction, cardiac dysfunction, or severe dyspnea, whereas a change from 97% at rest to 93% at peak exercise would not be expected to have important clinical consequences)
- Arterial blood gases may be measured in selected patients in order to provide more precise information about oxygenation as well as the partial pressure of carbon dioxide (P_aCO_2). In addition, the alveolar-arterial oxygen difference can be calculated to further evaluate gas exchange

---

SPECIFIC RESPIRATORY DISEASES

Asthma/COPD. Many patients with moderate to severe asthma or COPD exhibit abnormal cardiopulmonary exercise responses due to ventilatory limitations and/or oxygen desaturation. In patients in whom reactive airway disease is suspected or asthma has been documented, exercise-induced bronchoconstriction (EIB) frequently occurs. An exercise challenge test consisting of six to eight minutes of strenuous running on the treadmill at a target intensity of 85 to 90% of the maximal heart rate is frequently used to diagnose EIB. A positive test is a $\geq 15\%$ decrease in $FEV_{1.0}$ in the post-exercise period.

Interstitial lung disease. Oxygen desaturation is a common abnormality during exercise in patients with interstitial lung disease. In addition, these patients usually demonstrate evidence of ventilatory limitation as evidenced by a low BR.

Pulmonary vascular disease. Patients with pulmonary vascular disease typically exhibit a low BR, a low HR reserve, a high ventilatory equivalent for $\dot{V}CO_2$ ($\dot{V}_E/\dot{V}CO_2$ ratio), a low oxygen-pulse ($\dot{V}O_2/HR$), and oxygen desaturation.

Psychogenic dyspnea. The major abnormality is an irregular breathing pattern with fluctuating levels of ventilation. Psychogenic dyspnea is suspected if the patient performs at maximal effort, the BR is normal, and there is no evidence of oxygen desaturation.

Symptom limitation. Patients with moderate to severe respiratory disease usually report "severe" levels of dyspnea (e.g., 6 to 8 on the 1–10 category-ratio scale) at peak exercise. These perceptual responses are similar regardless of the specific disease. Assessing such patients using multiple subjective scales, e.g., comparative ratings of dyspnea and leg pain, may be useful for interpretation of the major limitation with respect to exercise. Some patients with respiratory disease who complain of "difficulty breathing with activities" may actually report higher ratings for leg discomfort/pain than dyspnea at submaximal and maximal exercise intensities. These results combined with a reduced $\dot{V}O_{2max}$ and a normal BR strongly suggest that the individual is limited by deconditioning and/or musculoskeletal factors rather than respiratory disease.

REFERENCES

1. Institute for Aerobics Research. Physical Fitness Norms. [Unpublished data reprinted with permission.] Dallas, TX, 1994.

2. Kemp HG, Kronmal RA, Vlietstra RE, and Frye FL: Seven year survival of patients with normal and near normal coronary arteriograms: a CASS registry study. *J Am Coll Cardiol* 7:479–483, 1986.

3. Siscovick DS, Ekelunch LG, Johnson JL, Trong Y, and Adler A: Sensitivity of exercise electrocardiography for acute cardiac events during moderate and strenuous physical activity. *Arch Int Med 151*:325–330, 1991.

4. Taylor HL, Buskirk ER, and Henschel A: Maximal oxygen uptake as an objective measure of cardiorespiratory performance. *J Appl Physiol 8*:73–80, 1955.

5. Londeree BR and Moeschberger ML: Influence of age and other factors on maximal heart rate. *J Cardiac Rehab 4*:44–49, 1984.

6. Wolthius RA, Froelicher VF, Fischer J, and Triebwasser JH: The response of healthy men to treadmill exercise. *Circulation 55*:153–157, 1977.

7. Weiner DA, McCabe CH, Cutler SS, and Ryan TJ: Decrease in systolic blood pressure during exercise testing: Reproducibility, response to coronary bypass surgery and prognostic significance. *Am J Cardiology. 49*:1627–1631, 1982.

8. Allison TG, Squires RW, and Gau GT: Maximal treadmill exercise blood pressure by age and gender. *Circulation 80*:240–246, 1989.

9. Myers J and Froelicher VF: Hemodynamic determinants of exercise capacity in chronic heart failure. *Ann Int Med 115*:377–386, 1991.

10. McKirnan MD, Sullivan M, Jensen D, and Froelicher VF: Treadmill performance and cardiac function in selected patients with coronary heart disease. *J Am Coll Cardiol* 3:253–261, 1984.

11. Hammond HK, Kelley TL, and Froelicher VF: Noninvasive testing in the evaluation of myocardial ischemia: Agreement among tests. *J Am Coll Cardiol* 5:59–69, 1985.

12. Myers J, Ahnve S, Froelicher V, and Sullivan M: Spatial R wave amplitude changes during exercise: Relation with left ventricular ischemia and function. *J Am Coll Cardiol* 6:603–608, 1985.

13. Mirvis DM, Ramanathan KB, and Wilson JL: Regional blood flow correlates of ST segment depression in tachycardia-induced myocardial ischemia. *Circulation* 2:363–373, 1986.

14. Nostratian F and Froelicher VF: ST elevation during exercise testing: a review. *Am J Cardiol* 63:986–988, 1989.

15. Lavie CJ. Oh JK, Mankin HT, Clements IP, Giuliani ER, and Gibbons RJ: Significance of T-wave pseudonormalization during exercise. A radionuclide angiographic study. *Chest* 94:512–516, 1988.

16. Lachterman B, Lehmann KG, Detrano R, et al: Comparison of ST segment: heart rate index to standard ST criteria for analysis of exercise electrocardiogram. *Circulation* 82:44–50, 1990.

17. Whinnery JE, Froelicher VF, and Stewart AJ: The electrocardiographic response to maximal treadmill exercise in asymptomatic men with left bundle branch block. *Am Heart J* 94:316, 1977

18. Vasey CG, O'Donnell J, Morris SN, and McHenry P: Exercise-induced left bundle branch block and its relation to coronary artery disease. *Am J Cardiol* 56:892–895, 1985.

19. Whinnery JE, Froelicher VF, and Stewart AJ: The electrocardiographic response to maximal treadmill exercise in asymptomatic men with right bundle branch block. *Chest* 71:335, 1977.

20. Busby MJ, Shefrin EA, and Fleg JL: Prevalence and long-term significance of exercise-induced frequent or repetitive ventricular ectopic beats in apparently healthy volunteers. *J Am Coll Cardiol* 14:1659–1665, 1989.

21. Yang JC, Wesley RC, and Froelicher VF: Ventricular tachycardia during routine treadmill testing. Risk and prognosis. *Arch Internal Med* 151:349–352, 1991.

22. Detrano R and Froelicher VF: Exercise testing: Uses and limitations considering recent studies. *Prog Cardiovasc Dis* *31*:173–204, 1988.

23. Fleg JL, Gerstenblith G, Zonderman AB, Becker LC, et al: Prevalence and prognostic significance of exercise-induced silent myocardial ischemia detected by thallium scintigraphy and electrocardiography in asymptomatic volunteers. *Circulation 81*:428–436, 1990.

24. Morrow K, Morris CK, Froelicher VF, Hideg A, et al: Prediction of cardiovascular death in men undergoing noninvasive evaluation for coronary artery disease. *Ann Int Med 118*(9), 1993.

25. Mark DB, Hlatky MA, Harrell FE, Lee KL, et al: Exercise treadmill score for predicting prognosis in coronary artery disease. *Ann Int Med 106*:793–800, 1987.

26. Hartz A, Gammaitoni C, and Young M: Quantitative analysis of the exercise tolerance test for determining the severity of coronary artery disease. *Int J Cardiol* 24:63–71, 1989.

section III

EXERCISE PRESCRIPTION

chapter 7

GENERAL PRINCIPLES OF EXERCISE PRESCRIPTION

INTRODUCTION

The essential components of a systematic, individualized exercise prescription include the appropriate mode(s), intensity, duration, frequency, and progression of physical activity. These five components apply when developing exercise prescriptions for persons of all ages and functional capacities, regardless of the presence or absence of risk factors and disease. The optimal exercise prescription for an individual is determined from an objective evaluation of that individual's response to exercise, including observations of heart rate (HR), blood pressure (BP), ratings of perceived exertion (RPE), subjective response to exercise, electrocardiogram (ECG) when applicable, and functional capacity measured during a graded exercise test (GXT). As discussed in Chapter 2, a GXT is not required for all individuals prior to beginning an exercise program. However, the exercise prescription should be developed with careful consideration of the individual's health status (including medications), risk factor profile, behavioral characteristics, personal goals, and exercise preferences.

PURPOSES OF THE EXERCISE PRESCRIPTION

Various purposes of exercise prescription include enhancing physical fitness, promoting health by reducing risk factors for chronic disease, and ensuring safety during exercise participation. Based on individual interests, health needs, and clinical status, these common purposes do not carry equal or consistent weight. In all cases, specific outcomes identified for a particular person should be the ultimate target of the exercise prescription.

When an exercise prescription is given by a non-licensed health care provider, it is important that the provider not independently present a prescription which would otherwise be utilized for the purposes of treating or alleviating disease or illness. Such prescriptions must necessarily be limited to those who are authorized by law to provide such recommendations. In practice, this typically translates into the co-signing of a prescription by a physician.

Traditional approaches to exercise prescription development have been based largely on the body of knowledge that links increased exercise participation to improved physical fitness, as measured by $\dot{V}O_{2max}$ and muscular performance. However, the quantity of exercise needed to significantly reduce disease risk appears to be considerably less than that needed to develop and maintain high levels of physical fitness. This observation carries important implications for health professionals, especially when improvement in health status for chronic disease is a primary patient outcome. For the sedentary person at risk for premature chronic disease, adoption of a moderately active lifestyle may carry important health benefits and represent a more attainable goal than achievement of a high $\dot{V}O_{2max}$. Regardless, enhancing physical fitness whenever possible is a desirable feature of exercise prescriptions.

THE ART OF EXERCISE PRESCRIPTION

The guidelines for exercise prescription presented in this book are based on a solid foundation of scientific information. Given the diverse nature and health needs of the population, these guidelines cannot be applied in an overly rigid or precise fashion, that is, by simply applying mathematical calculations based on test data. The techniques presented should be used with flexibility and with careful attention paid to the goals of the individual. Exercise prescriptions will require modification in accordance with observed individual responses and adaptations because:

- Physiological and perceptual responses to acute exercise vary
- Adaptations to exercise training vary in terms of magnitude and rate of development
- Desired outcomes based on individual need(s) may be obtained with exercise programs that vary considerably in their structure
- Behavioral adaptation to the exercise prescription is likewise quite variable

A fundamental objective of exercise prescription is to bring about a change in personal health behavior to include habitual physical activity. Thus, the most appropriate exercise prescription for a particular person is the one that is most helpful in achieving this behavioral change. *The art of exercise prescription is the successful integration of exercise science with behavioral techniques that result in long-term program compliance and attainment of the individual's goals.* As such, knowledge of methods to change health behaviors is essential. While there exists an abundance of literature on this topic, an excellent source is Section VIII of the *Resource Manual for Guidelines for Graded Exercise Testing and Prescription, 2nd ed.*

CARDIORESPIRATORY ENDURANCE

Improvement in the ability of the body to utilize oxygen efficiently, resulting in improved endurance, is one component of physical fitness. Improvement in cardiorespiratory fitness is measured by assessing change in maximal oxygen uptake ($\dot{V}O_{2max}$), which in turn is directly related to the frequency, duration, and intensity of exercise. Depending on the interaction of these prescriptive components, resultant increases in $\dot{V}O_{2max}$ may range from 5 to 30%. Individuals with low initial levels of fitness, cardiac patients, and those exhibiting large losses of body weight will demonstrate the greatest percent increase in $\dot{V}O_{2max}$. Similarly, more modest increases may be expected from healthy individuals with high initial levels of fitness and those who exhibit little change in body weight.

MODE OF EXERCISE

The greatest improvement in $\dot{V}O_{2max}$ occurs when exercise involves the use of large muscle groups over prolonged periods and is rhythmic and aerobic in nature (e.g. walking, hiking, running, machine-based stair climbing, swimming, cycling, rowing, combined arm and leg ergometry, dancing, skating, cross-country skiing, rope skipping, or endurance game activities). Clearly, this wide range of activities provides for individual variability relative to skill and enjoyment, factors which influence compliance to the exercise program and thus desired outcomes. Table 7–1 groups commonly prescribed activities. In the development of the exercise prescription for the novice exerciser, it may be useful to begin with Group 1 activities and progress depending on the individual's adaptation and clinical status. Resistive exercise such as weight training should not be considered as an activity for increasing $\dot{V}O_{2max}$ but is an important component of a sound overall exercise plan. Circuit weight training, which involves 10 to 15 repetitions with 15 to 30 seconds rest between weight stations, results in an average improvement in $\dot{V}O_{2max}$ of about 5%, and thus is not generally recommended as an activity for improving cardiorespiratory endurance.

TABLE 7–1. GROUPING OF CARDIORESPIRATORY ENDURANCE ACTIVITIES

Group 1   Activities that can be readily maintained at a constant intensity and interindividual variation in energy expenditure is relatively low. Desirable for more precise control of exercise intensity, as in the early stages of a rehabilitation program. Examples of these activities are walking and cycling, especially treadmill and cycle ergometry

Group 2   Activities where the rate of energy expenditure is highly related to skill, but for a given individual can provide a constant intensity. May also be useful in early stages of conditioning, but skill level must be considered. Examples include swimming and cross-country skiing

Group 3   Activities where both skill and intensity of exercise are highly variable. Such activities can be very useful to provide group interaction and variety in exercise, but must be cautiously considered for high-risk, low-fit, and/or symptomatic individuals. Competitive factors must also be considered and minimized. Examples of these activities are racquet sports and basketball

The risk of injury associated with high impact activities or high intensity weight training must also be weighed when selecting exercise modalities, especially for the novice exerciser or an obese individual. It may be desirable to engage in several different activities to reduce repetitive orthopedic stresses and involve a greater number of muscle groups. Because improvement in muscular endurance is largely specific to the muscles involved in exercise, it is important to consider unique vocational or recreational objectives of the exercise program when selecting activities. Finally, it is important to consider other barriers that might decrease the likelihood of compliance with, or adherence to, the exercise program (travel, cost, spousal or partner involvement, etc.).

EXERCISE INTENSITY

Intensity and duration of exercise determine the total caloric expenditure during a training session, and are integrally related. That is, similar increases in cardiorespiratory endurance may be achieved by a low intensity, long duration session as well as a higher intensity, shorter duration session. The risk of orthopedic injury may be increased with the latter; however, programs emphasizing low- to moderate-intensity exercise with a longer training duration are recommended for most individuals. ACSM recommends that the intensity of exercise be prescribed as 60 to 90% of maximum heart rate (HR_{max}), or 50 to 85% of $\dot{V}O_{2max}$ or HR reserve.[1] However, individuals with a very low initial level of fitness respond to a low exercise intensity, for example, 40 to 50% of $\dot{V}O_{2max}$.

Several important factors to consider prior to determining the level of exercise intensity include:

- Individual's level of fitness
- Presence of medications that may influence heart rate
- Risk of cardiovascular or orthopedic injury
- Individual preferences for exercise
- Individual program objectives

HR methods. Using HR as a guide to exercise intensity is useful, given the relatively linear relationship between HR and $\dot{V}O_2$. Because maximal HR (HR_{max}) declines with age and has large inter-individual differences (see Appendix D), it is best to measure HR_{max} during a maximal graded exercise test whenever possible. When prescribing exercise intensity based on HR, consideration must be given to potential influences. For example, medications such as β-blocking agents will reduce resting HR and the HR response to exercise (specific cardiodynamic effects of medications may be found in Appendix A). During an actual exercise session, the assumption exists that the individual will achieve a steady state HR response in the prescribed range; in reality (and certainly during discontinuous exercise) HR is likely to be both above and below prescribed range. The goal should be to maintain an average HR close to the midpoint of the prescribed range.

Given exercise test data, there are several approaches to determining an exercise HR range for prescriptive purposes:

- Using a straight percentage of HR_{max}
- Using the HR reserve method
- Plotting HR vs. VO_2 or exercise intensity during the exercise test

The assumption is made that 60 to 90% of HR_{max} is equivalent to 50 to 85% of $\dot{V}O_{2max}$ or HR reserve.[1] If an individual's HR_{max} is 180, the target HR range would be 108 (60%) to 162 (90%) beats/minute. The HR reserve method (Karvonen formula) is demonstrated below:

- Subtract standing resting heart rate (HR_{rest}) from maximal heart rate (HR_{max}) to obtain heart rate reserve
- Calculate 50% and 85% of the heart rate reserve
- Add each of these values to resting HR to obtain the target HR range, e.g.:
    Target HR range = $[(HR_{max} - HR_{rest}) \times 0.50$ and $0.85]$ $+ HR_{rest}$

Assuming an HR_{rest} of 60 beats/min, this latter method yields a target HR range of 120 to 162 beats/min.

A third method involves plotting HR against either measured $\dot{V}O_2$ (Figure 7–1) or exercise intensity (as discussed in Chapter 4). If RPE data have also been collected, the HR-$\dot{V}O_2$ relationship can be further evaluated in relation to the individual's RPE, which is helpful in assessing intensity during exercise. Plotting data better depicts the interrelationships between HR, $\dot{V}O_2$, and RPE and results in a more appropriate exercise intensity for persons with limited skills, those who held handrails during the GXT, and those with various diseases and medication effects. When plotting is not feasible, Table 7–2 provides approximate relationships among these variables, based on 30 to 60 minutes of exercise.[2]

RPE. Commonly used RPE scales are found in Chapter 4. Use of RPE should be considered as an adjunct to monitoring HR, as RPE determined during a GXT may not consistently translate directly to the same intensity during an exercise session. A small percentage of individuals

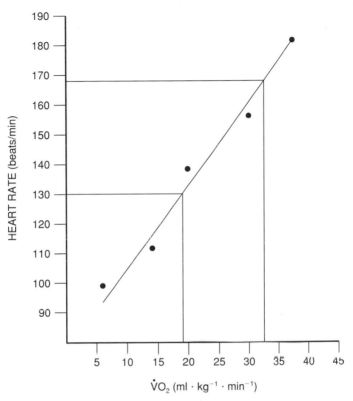

FIG. 7–1. A line of best fit has been drawn through the data points on this plot of heart rate and oxygen consumption data observed during a hypothetical maximal exercise test in which $\dot{V}O_{2max}$ was observed to be 38 ml · kg^{-1}· min^{-1} and maximal heart rate was 184 beats/min. A target heart rate range was determined by finding the heart rates that correspond to 50% and 85% of $\dot{V}O_{2max}$. For this individual, 50% of $\dot{V}O_{2max}$ was approximately 19 ml · kg^{-1}· min^{-1} and 85% of $\dot{V}O_{2max}$ was approximately 32 ml · kg^{-1}· min^{-1}. The corresponding heart rates are approximately 130 and 168 beats/min. The target heart rate range for this individual is 130 to 168 beats/min.

TABLE 7–2. CLASSIFICATION OF INTENSITY OF EXERCISE BASED ON 30 TO 60 MINUTES OF ENDURANCE TRAINING*

% HR_{max}	% $\dot{V}O_{2max}$	RPE	Classification of Intensity
<35	<30	<10	Very light
35–59	30–49	10–11	Light
60–79	50–74	12–13	Moderate
80–89	75–84	14–16	Heavy
>90	>85	>16	Very heavy

*Reprinted with permission from Reference 2.

(~10%) are unable to reliably use the scale. However, it has proven to be a valuable aid in prescribing exercise for individuals who have difficulty with HR palpation, and in cases where the HR response to exercise may have been altered due to a change in medication, provided a repeat graded exercise test is not performed. The RPE range associated with physiological adaptation to exercise is 12 to 16 (somewhat hard to hard) on the original Borg scale (Table 7–2).

METs. The energy costs of various physical activities have been extensively studied. Table 7–3 lists a variety of these activities and may be useful in initial consideration of these activities when developing the exercise prescription. For Group 1 activities listed in Table 7–1, the metabolic calculations found in these *Guidelines* will assist in estimating the MET costs for varying activity intensities. There is considerable variability in actual MET costs for Group 2 and Group 3 activities and it is necessary to clarify the intensity with the individual and monitor intensity closely. Prescribing by METs is most logically applicable to the apparently healthy and those with high $\dot{V}O_{2max}$ values. It is less applicable for individuals with cardiac or pulmonary disease, or for individuals with low functional capacities.

Integration of data. Several acceptable methods are

available for determining the appropriate exercise intensity. Accurate assessment of hemodynamic, metabolic, and perceptual responses to exercise provides adequate information for exercise prescription. Ancillary data, such as ventilatory threshold or blood lactate threshold, permit further evaluation for clinical purposes. In the final analysis, the appropriate exercise intensity is one that is safe, tolerable, and achieves the desired caloric output given the time constraints of the exercise session.

EXERCISE DURATION

The time constraints imposed on the individual influence both the duration and frequency of exercise sessions. Although improvements in cardiorespiratory endurance have been demonstrated with 5 to 10 minutes of very high intensity (>90% $\dot{V}O_{2max}$) exercise, the risk-benefit tradeoff of this format argues against its consideration. Typically, caloric goals can be best met in sessions lasting 20 to 30 minutes, excluding time spent warming up and cooling down. ACSM recommends 20 to 60 minutes of continuous aerobic activity.[1] Initial goals should be set reasonably so that individuals can reach preset goals with exercise sessions of moderate duration (20 to 30 minutes). For severely deconditioned individuals, multiple sessions of short duration (~10 minutes) may be necessary. Increases in exercise duration should be instituted as the individual adapts to training without evidence of undue fatigue or injury. The rate of progression in exercise is discussed later in the chapter.

EXERCISE FREQUENCY

Frequency is interrelated with both intensity and duration of exercise and therefore depends on those two variables. However, functional capacity is of key importance. Patients with functional capacities of <3 METs benefit

TABLE 7–3. LEISURE ACTIVITIES IN METs: SPORTS, EXERCISE CLASSES, GAMES, DANCING

	Mean	Range
Archery	3.9	3–4
Backpacking	—	5–11
Badminton	5.8	4–9+
Basketball		
Gameplay	8.3	7–12+
Non-game	—	3–9
Billiards	2.5	—
Bowling	—	2–4
Boxing		
In-ring	13.3	—
Sparring	8.3	—
Canoeing, rowing, and kayaking	—	3–8
Conditioning exercise	—	3–8+
Climbing hills	7.2	5–10+
Cricket	5.2	4–8
Croquet	3.5	—
Cycling		
Pleasure or to work	—	3–8+
10 mph	7.0	—
Dancing (social, square, tap)	—	3–8
Dancing (aerobic)	—	6–9
Fencing	—	6–10+
Field hockey	8.0	—
Fishing		
From bank	3.7	2–4
Wading in stream	—	5–6
Football (touch)	7.9	6–10
Golf		
Power cart	—	2–3
Walking (carrying bag or pulling cart)	5.1	4–7
Handball	—	8–12+
Hiking (cross-country)	—	3–7
Horseback riding		
Galloping	8.2	—
Trotting	6.6	—
Walking	2.4	—

Continued on Next Page

TABLE 7–3. *Continued*

	Mean	Range
Horseshoe pitching	—	2–3
Hunting (bow or gun)		
Small game (walking, carrying light load)	—	3–7
Big game (dragging carcass, walking)	—	3–14
Judo	13.5	—
Mountain climbing	—	5–10+
Music playing	—	2–3
Paddleball, racquetball	9	8–12
Rope jumping	11	—
60–80 skips/min	9	—
120–140 skips/min	—	11–12
Running		
12 min per mile	8.7	—
11 min per mile	9.4	—
10 min per mile	10.2	—
9 min per mile	11.2	—
8 min per mile	12.5	—
7 min per mile	14.1	—
6 min per mile	16.3	—
Sailing	—	2–5
Scuba diving	—	5–10
Shuffleboard	—	2–3
Skating, ice and roller	—	5–8
Skiing, snow		
Downhill	—	5–8
Cross country	—	6–12+
Skiing, water	—	5–7
Sledding, tobogganing	—	4–8
Snowshoeing	9.9	7–14
Squash	—	8–12+
Soccer	—	5–12+
Stair climbing	—	4–8
Swimming	—	4–8+
Table tennis	4.1	3–5
Tennis	6.5	4–9+
Volleyball	—	3–6

from multiple short daily exercise sessions; one to two sessions/day are most appropriate for three to five MET capacities; and 3 to 5 sessions/week are recommended for individuals with functional capacities >5 METs. Clearly, the number of exercise sessions per week will vary given caloric goals, participant preferences, and limitations imposed by the participant's lifestyle.

CALORIC THRESHOLDS FOR ADAPTATION

The interaction of intensity, duration, and frequency determines caloric expenditure. The thresholds necessary to bring about significant improvement in $\dot{V}O_{2max}$, weight loss, or reduced risk of premature chronic disease may be different. Since reduction of body weight (or body fatness) is a frequently desired outcome in exercise programs, considerable research has been directed to ascertaining the appropriate volume of activity necessary to reduce adiposity. ACSM recommends *minimal* thresholds of 300 kcal per exercise session performed 3 days per week, or 200 kcal per session done 4 days per week.[1] This suggests a weekly threshold of 800 to 900 exercise kcals per week, which is somewhat less than the recommendation in the previous edition of the Guidelines. It would appear that a reasonable approach in prescribed exercise programs is to target a weekly exercise caloric expenditure of approximately 1000 kcal. To achieve optimal physical activity levels the goal is to bring the weekly expenditure closer to 2000 kcal as health and fitness permits.

Estimating caloric expenditure during exercise has been problematic for exercise professionals and developing an exercise plan based on caloric thresholds has posed difficulties. As discussed previously, interindividual differences in skill, coordination, and exercise economy (the $\dot{V}O_2$ at a given submaximal work rate) and the variable intensities within each available activity strongly influence estimation of caloric expenditure during exercise. One useful method to approximate the caloric cost of exercise is by using the following equation based on the MET level of the activity:

$$\text{METs} \times 3.5 \times \text{body weight in kg} / 200 = \text{kcal/min}$$

This formula has utility in helping an individual understand the components of the exercise prescription and the volume of exercise necessary to achieve the caloric goals of the program. For example, if the weekly goal of the program has been set at 1000 calories, the individual weighs 70 kg, and the MET level of the prescribed activity is 6 METS, the caloric expenditure is 7.35 kcal/min, requiring 136 minutes per week. Given a 3 day per week program, the individual will require 45 minutes per day to achieve the 1000 kcal goal (or 34 minutes per day, 4 days per week). Working backward from the caloric goal to determine the volume of exercise needed to reach the goal is useful in determining the appropriate exercise prescription components.

RATE OF PROGRESSION

The recommended rate of progression in an exercise conditioning program depends on functional capacity, medical and health status, age, and individual activity preferences and goals. For apparently healthy adults, the endurance aspect of the exercise prescription has 3 stages

TABLE 7-4. EXAMPLE: PROGRESSION OF THE PRESUMABLY HEALTHY PARTICIPANT

Program Phase	Wk	Exercise Frequency (Sessions/Wk)	Exercise Intensity (% $\dot{V}O_{2max}$ or HR Reserve)	Exercise Duration (min)
Initial Stage	1	3	40–50	12
	2	3	50	14
	3	3	60	16
	4	3	60–70	18
	5	3	60–70	20
Improvement Stage	6–9	3–4	70–80	21
	10–13	3–4	70–80	24
	14–16	3–4	70–80	24
	17–19	4–5	70–80	28
	20–23	4–5	70–80	30
	24–27	4–5	70–85	30
Maintenance Stage	28+	3	70–85	30–45

of progression: initial, improvement, and maintenance (see Table 7–4).

INITIAL CONDITIONING STAGE

The initial stage should include light muscular endurance exercises and low level aerobic activities (40 to 60% of HR reserve or $\dot{V}O_{2max}$), exercises which are compatible with minimal muscle soreness, discomfort, and injury. Exercise adherence may decrease if the program is too aggressively initiated. This stage usually lasts 4 to 6 weeks, but the length depends on the adaptation of the individual to the exercise program. The duration of the exercise session during the initial stage should begin with approximately 12 to 15 minutes and progress to 20 minutes. It is recommended that individuals who are starting a conditioning program exercise three times per week on non-consecutive days.

Individual goals should be established early in the exercise program. They should be developed by the participant with the guidance of an exercise professional. The goals must be realistic and a system of rewards—intrinsic or extrinsic—should be established at that time.

IMPROVEMENT STAGE

The improvement stage of the exercise conditioning program differs from the initial stage in that the participant is progressed at a more rapid rate. This stage typically lasts 4 to 5 months, during which intensity is progressively increased within the upper half of the target range of 50 to 85% $\dot{V}O_{2max}$. Duration is increased consistently every 2 to 3 weeks until participants are able to exercise for 20 to 30 minutes continuously. The frequency and magnitude of the increments are dictated by the rate at which the participant adapts to the conditioning program. Deconditioned individuals should be permitted more time for adaptation at each stage of conditioning. Age should also be taken into consideration when progressions are recommended, as experience suggests that adaptation to conditioning may take longer in older individuals.

MAINTENANCE STAGE

The maintenance stage of the exercise program usually begins after the first six months of training. During this stage the participant may no longer be interested in further increasing the conditioning stimulus. Further improvement may be minimal, but continuing the same workout routine enables individuals to maintain their fitness levels.

At this point, the goals of the program should be reviewed and new goals set. To maintain fitness, a specific exercise program should be designed that will be similar in energy cost to the conditioning program and satisfy the needs and interests of the participant over an extended period. It is important to include exercises that the individual finds enjoyable.

MUSCULOSKELETAL FLEXIBILITY

Optimal musculoskeletal function requires that an adequate range of motion be maintained in all joints. Of particular importance is maintenance of flexibility in the lower back and posterior thigh regions. Lack of flexibility in this area may be associated with an increased risk for the development of chronic lower back pain. Therefore, preventive and rehabilitative exercise programs should include activities that promote the maintenance of flexibility. Lack of flexibility is prevalent in the elderly among whom this condition often contributes to a reduced ability to perform activities of daily living (ADL). Accordingly, exercise programs for the elderly should emphasize proper stretching, especially for the upper and lower trunk, neck, and hip regions.

There are different types of stretching techniques [e.g., static, ballistic, and proprioceptive neuromuscular facilitation (PNF)] that can be performed. Static stretching involves slowly stretching a muscle to the point of mild discomfort and then holding that position for an extended period of time (usually 10 to 30 seconds). The risk of injury is low, it requires little time and assistance, and is quite effective. For these reasons, static stretching is the most commonly recommended method. Ballistic stretching uses the momentum created by repetitive bouncing movements to produce muscle stretch. This type of stretch can result in muscle soreness or injury if the forces generated by the ballistic movements are too great. PNF stretching involves a combination of alternating contraction and relaxation of both agonist and antagonist muscles. While research has suggested that PNF stretching produces the largest improvements in flexibility, this technique typically causes some degree of muscle soreness. Moreover, it typically requires a partner and is more time-consuming than alternative techniques.

Properly performed stretching exercises can aid in improving and maintaining range of motion in a joint or series of joints. Flexibility exercises should be performed in a slow, controlled manner with a gradual progression to greater ranges of motion. A general exercise prescription for achieving and maintaining flexibility should adhere to the following guidelines:

• Frequency:	At least 3 days per week
• Intensity:	To a position of mild discomfort
• Duration:	10 to 30 seconds for each stretch
• Repetitions:	3 to 5 for each stretch
• Type:	Static, with a major emphasis on the lower back and thigh area

A series of easy-to-understand stretches are published in the *ACSM Fitness Book.* Stretching exercises can be effectively included in the warm-up and/or cool-down periods that precede and follow the aerobic conditioning phase of an exercise session. It is recommended that an active warm-up precede vigorous stretching exercises. Some commonly employed stretching exercises may not be appropriate for some participants who may—through prior injury, joint insufficiency, or other condition—be at greater risk for musculoskeletal injuries. Although research evidence concerning the risks of specific exercises is lacking, those activities that require substantial flexibility and/or skill are not recommended for older, less flexible, and less experienced participants.

MUSCULAR FITNESS

Although aerobic activities have been shown to be effective for developing cardiorespiratory fitness, most have little influence on muscular strength or muscular endurance, especially of the upper body. Every activity— including ADL—requires a certain percentage of an individual's maximal strength and endurance. The maintenance or enhancement of muscular strength and muscular endurance enables an individual to perform such tasks with less physiological stress. The physiological stress induced by lifting or holding a given weight is proportional to the percentage of maximal strength involved.

Resistance training of moderate intensity (i.e, sufficient to develop and maintain muscular fitness and lean body weight) should be an integral part of adult fitness and rehabilitative exercise programs. In addition to the development and maintenance of muscular strength and muscle mass, the physiological benefits of resistance training include increases in bone mass and in the strength of connective tissue. These adaptations are beneficial for middle-age and older adults, and, in particular, postmenopausal women who rapidly lose bone mineral density. Other health benefits which have been ascribed to resistance training include: modest improvements in cardiorespiratory fitness, reductions in body fat, modest reductions in blood pressure, improved glucose tolerance, and improved blood lipid and lipoprotein profiles. These health benefits have been most often associated with circuit weight training, which is a method of resistance training in which a series of exercises are performed in succession with minimal rest between exercises.

Muscular strength and endurance are developed by the overload principle—by increasing the resistance to movement or the frequency or duration of activity to levels above those normally experienced. Muscular strength is best developed by using weights that develop maximal or nearly maximal muscle tension with relatively few repetitions. Muscular endurance is best developed by using lighter weights with a greater number of repetitions. To elicit improvement in both muscular strength and endurance, most experts recommend 8 to 12 repetitions per exercise.

Any overload will result in strength development, but higher intensity effort at or near maximal effort will produce a significantly greater effect. The intensity of resistance training can be manipulated by varying the weight, the number of repetitions, the length of the rest interval between exercises, or the number of sets of exercises completed. Caution is advised for training that emphasizes lengthening (eccentric) contractions, compared to shortening (concentric) or isometric contractions, as the potential for skeletal muscle soreness is accentuated.

Muscular strength and endurance can be developed by means of static or dynamic exercises. Although each type of training has strengths and weaknesses, dynamic resistance exercises are recommended for most adults. Resistance training for the average participant should be rhythmical, performed at a moderate-to-slow speed, involve a full range of motion, and not interfere with normal breathing. Heavy resistance exercise combined with breath-holding can cause a dramatic, acute increase in both systolic and diastolic blood pressure (Valsalva maneuver).

The following resistance training guidelines are recommended for the apparently healthy adult:

- Perform a minimum of 8 to 10 separate exercises that train the major muscle groups
  A primary goal of the program should be to develop total body strength in a relatively time-efficient manner. Programs lasting longer than 1 hour per session are associated with higher dropout rates.
- Perform one set of 8 to 12 repetitions of each of these exercises to the point of volitional fatigue
- Perform these exercises at least 2 days per week
  While more frequent training and additional sets or combinations of sets and repetitions elicit larger strength gains, the additional improvement is relatively small
- Adhere as closely as possible to the specific techniques for performing a given exercise
- Perform every exercise through a full range of motion

- Perform both the lifting (concentric phase) and lowering (eccentric phase) portion of the resistance exercises in a controlled manner
- Maintain a normal breathing pattern, since breath-holding can induce excessive increases in blood pressure
- If possible, exercise with a training partner who can provide feedback, assistance, and motivation

PROGRAM SUPERVISION

Information from health screening, medical evaluation, and exercise testing allow the exercise professional to determine those individuals for whom supervised exercise programs are suggested. Table 7–5 provides criteria for participation in unsupervised versus supervised programs.

Supervised exercise programs are particularly recommended for symptomatic and cardiorespiratory disease patients who are considered by their physicians to be clinically stable and who have been cleared by their physicians for participation in such programs. It is recom-

TABLE 7–5. GENERAL GUIDELINES FOR PARTICIPATION IN UNSUPERVISED AND SUPERVISED EXERCISE PROGRAMS

	Program	
	Unsupervised	Supervised
Health status	Apparently healthy	Two or more major CAD risk factors Known CAD
Functional capacity	≥8 METs	<8 METs*

*For functional capacity <5 METS, a small staff-to-patient ratio (i.e., one professional staff member for every 5 to 8 patients) is also recommended.

mended that supervised exercise programs be under the combined overall guidance of a physician and an ACSM-certified Program Director$_{SM}$ or Exercise Specialist$_{SM}$. Direct supervision of each session by a physician is, however, not required. These programs can be useful for those who need instruction in proper exercise techniques. For some participants, direct supervision may enhance compliance with an exercise program.

REFERENCES

1. ACSM. The recommended quantity and quality of exercise for developing and maintaining cardiorespiratory and muscular fitness in healthy adults. (Position Stand of the American College of Sports Medicine). *Med Sci Sports Exerc* 22:265–274, 1990.
2. Pollock ML and Wilmore JH: *Exercise in Health and Disease: Evaluation and Prescription for Prevention and Rehabilitation,* 2nd Ed. Philadelphia: WB Saunders, 1990.

chapter 8

EXERCISE PRESCRIPTION FOR CARDIAC PATIENTS

Properly prescribed exercise during hospitalization and following discharge affords numerous benefits for appropriately selected patients, in addition to those mentioned in Chapter 1:

- Offset the deleterious psychological and physiological effects of bed rest
- Provide additional medical surveillance of patients
- Identify patients with significant cardiovascular, physical, or cognitive impairments that may influence safety
- Enable patients to return to activities of daily living within the limits imposed by their disease
- Prepare the patient and the support system at home to optimize recovery following hospital discharge

Programs have traditionally been categorized as Phase I (inpatient), Phase II (up to 12 weeks of continuous ECG telemetry following discharge), Phase III (variable length program of intermittent or no ECG monitoring under supervision) and Phase IV (no ECG monitoring, limited supervision). New theories of risk stratification, recent data on the safety of exercise, and pressures of health care reform have contributed to a change in traditional cardiac rehabilitation services. There is now movement toward a structure wherein patients follow a regimen of exercise specific to their vocational and recreational needs, with more individualization of the length of program, degree of ECG monitoring, and level of clinical supervision. Such recommendations have been published in the literature[1,2] and form the bases for the risk stratification models presented in Chapter 2.

INPATIENT PROGRAMS

Clinical indications for cardiac rehabilitation are listed in Table 8–1. While not all patients in these categories may be suitable candidates for inpatient exercise, virtually all will benefit from some level of inpatient intervention, including risk factor modification, activity counseling, and patient and family education. Because of the decreased length of hospital stay for most cardiac patients, traditional programs with multiple steps for increasing activity are no longer feasible. In many instances, patients are now seen for only 3 to 7 days following referral to an inpatient cardiac rehabilitation program. Assessment of functional tolerance to activities of daily living, an emphasis on patient activity counseling and education have become major components of inpatient cardiac rehabilitation.

Inpatients should be risk-stratified as early as possible following hospitalization. The AACVPR or ACP risk stratification models[1,3] (Chapter 2) are useful for inpatients, as they include clinical criteria not included in other risk

TABLE 8-1. CLINICAL INDICATIONS AND CONTRAINDICATIONS FOR INPATIENT AND OUTPATIENT CARDIAC REHABILITATION

Indications

1. Medically stable post-MI
2. Stable angina
3. Coronary artery bypass graft (CABG) surgery
4. Percutaneous transluminal coronary angioplasty (PTCA)
5. Compensated congestive heart failure (CHF)
6. Cardiomyopathy
7. Heart or other organ transplantation
8. Other cardiac surgery including valvular and pacemaker insertion [including automatic implantable cardioverter defibrillator (AICD)]
9. Peripheral vascular disease
10. High-risk cardiovascular disease ineligible for surgical intervention
11. Sudden cardiac death syndrome
12. End-stage renal disease
13. At risk for CAD, with diagnoses of diabetes mellitus, hyperlipidemia, hypertension, etc.
14. Other patients who may benefit from structured exercise and/or patient education (based on physician referral and consensus of the rehabilitation team)

Contraindications

1. Unstable angina
2. Resting SBP >200 mm Hg or resting DBP >110 mm Hg should be evaluated on a case-by-case basis
3. Orthostatic blood pressure drop of >20 mm Hg with symptoms
4. Critical aortic stenosis (peak systolic pressure gradient >50 mm Hg with aortic valve orifice area <0.75 cm^2 in average size adult)
5. Acute systemic illness or fever
6. Uncontrolled atrial or ventricular arrhythmias
7. Uncontrolled sinus tachycardia (>120 beats/min)
8. Uncompensated CHF
9. 3° AV block (without pacemaker)
10. Active pericarditis or myocarditis
11. Recent embolism
12. Thrombophlebitis
13. Resting ST segment displacement (>2 mm)
14. Uncontrolled diabetes (resting blood glucose >400 mg/dl)
15. Severe orthopedic problems that would prohibit exercise
16. Other metabolic problems, such as acute thyroiditis, hypo- or hyperkalemia, hypovolemia, etc.

stratification models. Contraindications to entry into inpatient programs are included in Table 8–1, although exceptions should be considered based on sound clinical judgment. In addition to these contraindications, certain clinical characteristics appear to increase the risk of exercise-related complications (see Chapter 2). Table 8–2 details complicating factors following myocardial infarction to assist the clinician in identifying the high-risk inpatient population.[4] Pre-morbid status and course of hospitalization will influence the patient's functional status, perhaps on a daily basis.

Activities during the first 48 hours following MI and/or cardiac surgery should logically be restricted to self-care activities, arm and leg range of motion movement, and other low-resistance activities. The posture in which these activities are performed should progress from lying to sitting to standing. Where available, the use of treadmills and other ergometers is highly recommended for uncomplicated patients, usually 3 to 5 days postevent, as it provides more precise quantification in the assessment of exercise tolerance. As a means to further assist the clinician, Table 8–3 suggests a functional classification guide. In general, the criteria for terminating an exercise session are similar to those for terminating an exercise test (Table 5–4).

TABLE 8–2. COMPLICATING FACTORS AFTER MYOCARDIAL INFARCTION

Low-risk patients	• No complicating factors by day 4
Moderate-risk patients	• Poor ventricular function (EF <30%), or
	• Significant ischemia with low-level (2-3 MET) activity beyond day 4
High-risk patients	• Continued ischemia
	• Left ventricular failure
	• Episode of shock
	• Serious arrhythmias

TABLE 8-3. FUNCTIONAL CLASSIFICATION GUIDE FOR INPATIENT ACTIVITIES

Functional Class I	Functional Class II	Functional Class III
Sits up in bed with assistance Does own self-care activities—seated, or may need assistance Stands at bedside with assistance Sits up in chair 15 to 30 minutes, 2 to 3 times per day	Sits up in bed independently Stands independently Does self-care activities in bathroom—seated Walks in room and to bathroom (may need assistance)	Sits and stands independently Does own self-care activities in bathroom, seated or standing Walks in halls with assistance short distances (50 to 100 ft) as tolerated, up to 3 times per day
Functional Class IV	**Functional Class V**	**Functional Class VI**
Does own self-care and bathes Walks in halls short distances (150 to 200 ft) with minimal assistance, 3 to 4 times per day	Walks in halls independently, moderate distances (250 to 500 ft), 3 to 4 times per day.	Independent ambulation on unit 3 to 6 times per day

The optimal dosage of exercise for inpatients depends in part on medical history, clinical status, and symptoms. Upper limits to exercise should be physician-directed. For patients who are asymptomatic and do not demonstrate ischemia during exercise, the ability to tolerate exercise is more important than exercise HR as an indicator of appropriate intensity (HR guidelines for inpatients may not be possible in the absence of prior exercise evaluation). However, several general criteria may be used:

Intensity
- RPE <13 (6–20 scale)
- Post-MI: HR <120 beats/min or HR_{rest} + 20 beats/min (arbitrary targets)
- Post-surgery: HR_{rest} + 30 beats/min (arbitrary target)
- To tolerance if asymptomatic

Duration
- Intermittent bouts lasting 3–5 min
- Rest periods
  - at patient's discretion
  - lasting 1–2 min
  - shorter than exercise bout duration
- Total duration of up to 20 min

Frequency
- Early mobilization: 3–4 times per day (days 1–3)
- Later mobilization: 2 times per day (beginning on day 3)

Progression
- Initially increase duration to 10–15 min of continuous exercise, then increase intensity

---

By hospital discharge, a general goal is an exercise capacity of 5 METs, although this may be overly ambitious for many patients. Discharge functional capacity may be assessed by a GXT or by performance of activities approximating 4 to 5 METs, such as stair-climbing. Prior to discharge the patient should demonstrate a knowledge of those activities that are inappropriate or excessive and a safe, progressive plan of exercise and optimal risk reduction should be formulated for patients to take home. The patient should also be made aware of outpatient exercise program options and be provided with information regarding the use of home exercise equipment. Patients should be able to manage their rehabilitation independently and report cardiovascular symptoms promptly, should they occur.

OUTPATIENT PROGRAMS

Presuming that the goals for inpatient cardiac rehabilitation are met, the goals for outpatient programs are to:

- Provide appropriate patient supervision to ensure detection of problems and potential complications and provide timely feedback to the referring physician in order to enhance effective medical management
- Contingent on patient clinical status, return the patient to pre-morbid vocational and/or recreational activities, modify these activities as necessary, or find alternate activities
- Develop and help the patient implement a safe and effective home exercise program and recreational lifestyle
- Provide patient and family education to maximize secondary prevention

The implementation of a risk stratification model permits classification of patients according to their subsequent risk of death or cardiovascular complication (based on 1- and 5-year mortality and morbidity data). Risk stratification, however, should be only one factor to consider when making recommendations for outpatient supervision and the extent of ECG telemetry monitoring of cardiac patients.

Chapter 7 details various prescriptive techniques for determining the amount of exercise, that is, frequency, intensity, and duration. Plotting the exercise test data is recommended whenever possible, so that the relationships among $\dot{V}O_2$, HR, and RPE can be ascertained. For many cardiac patients, it is also critical to know when myocardial ischemia occurs during exercise, so that the patient can exercise below the anginal or ischemic threshold. A peak exercise HR 10 beats/minute below the threshold is generally appropriate. Table 8–4 outlines criteria for setting a safe upper limit for exercise intensity in cardiac patients. It is also important to consider medication effects and those clinical characteristics that place the patient at increased risk for a cardiovascular event (see Appendix A).

Whenever possible, patients should be encouraged to engage in multiple activities to promote total physical

---

TABLE 8–4. SIGNS AND SYMPTOMS BELOW WHICH AN UPPER LIMIT FOR EXERCISE INTENSITY SHOULD BE SET*

1. Onset of angina or other symptoms of cardiovascular insufficiency
2. Plateau or decrease in systolic blood pressure, systolic blood pressure >240 mm Hg, or diastolic blood pressure >110 mm Hg
3. >1 mm ST- segment depression, horizontal or downsloping
4. Radionuclide evidence of LV dysfunction or onset of moderate to severe wall motion abnormalities during exertion
5. Increased frequency of ventricular arrhythmias
6. Other significant ECG disturbances (e.g., 2° or 3° AV block, atrial fibrillation, SVT, complex ventricular ectopy, etc.)
7. Other signs/symptoms of intolerance to exercise

*The peak exercise HR should be approximately 10 beats/min below the HR associated with any of the above criteria.

conditioning, including appropriate resistance training. Where possible, use of a variety of equipment (treadmills, cycle and arm ergometers, stair-climbers, and rowing machines) is encouraged to maximize the carry-over of training benefits to real-life activities.

OUTPATIENT RATE OF PROGRESSION

While patients present for outpatient cardiac rehabilitation with a wide range of functional capacities, it is important to individualize exercise progression. It is generally prudent to progress patients to a level of exercise that will elicit a minimal caloric output of approximately 1000 kcal/week, at a mild to moderate exercise intensity. Progression has been traditionally divided into an initial conditioning phase, followed by improvement and maintenance stages. General principles for progressing the patient include an increase in exercise (as tolerated by the patient) every 1 to 3 weeks, with a goal of achieving 20 to 30 minutes of continuous exercise before prescribing additional increases in intensity. Patients requiring an intermittent format, such as those with PVD, should be progressed according to symptoms and clinical status. Intensity should be kept low until a continuous duration of 10 to 15 minutes is achieved. An example of exercise progression using an intermittent format is presented in Table 8–5. The progression should be guided by goals associated with the vocational and recreational needs within the limits imposed by disease.

A goal at the time of hospital discharge for most patients is a functional capacity >5 METs, which permits safe participation in most activities at home. Patients with lower functional capacities have a poorer prognosis and require a more conservative approach to exercise therapy, and thus progress more slowly. Conversely, patients with higher functional capacities respond well to more rapid progression. Fortunately, patients with low functional capacities respond favorably to lower intensity activity emphasizing frequent short bouts of exercise with intermittent rest periods. Because they often have impaired cardiac function, the emphasis for adaptation shifts to peripheral mechanisms. An example of a progression from intermittent to continuous exercise is found in Table 8–5. It is important to individualize the exercise prescription based on clinical status and symptoms. Consideration should be given to other factors that could hinder long-term adherence, compliance, and exercise progression, such as orthopedic problems.

TABLE 8–5. EXAMPLE OF EXERCISE PROGRESSION USING INTERMITTENT EXERCISE

A. FUNCTIONAL CAPACITY (FC) >3 METs

Wk	%FC	Total Min at %FC	Min Exercise	Min Rest	Reps
1	50–60	15–20	3–5	3–5	3–4
2	50–60	15–20	7–10	2–3	3
3	60–70	20–30	10–15	Optional	2
4	60–70	30–40	15–20	Optional	2

B. FC <3 METS

Wk	%FC	Total Min at %FC	Min Exercise	Min Rest	Reps
1	40–50	10–15	3–5	3–5	3–4
2	40–50	12–20	5–7	3–5	3
3	50–60	15–25	7–10	3–5	3
4	50–60	20–30	10–15	2–3	2
5	60–70	25–40	12–20	2	2
6	Continue with two reps of continuous exercise, with one rest period or progress to a single continuous bout				

TYPES OF OUTPATIENT PROGRAMS

For most patients, progression toward an independent self-managed program is desirable, but some patients may need to remain in a clinically supervised program. These include patients at high risk for cardiovascular complications, those unable to self-monitor, or those whose adherence depends heavily on group support. As a general rule, most patients should participate in a clinically supervised rehabilitation program for at least 3 months to facilitate both exercise and lifestyle management changes. Clinically supervised programs have traditionally been divided into Phase II and Phase III, both of which are supervised by a clinically trained staff. Given the shifting parameters for classifying cardiac patients and prescrib-

TABLE 8–6. GUIDELINES FOR PROGRESSION TO INDEPENDENT EXERCISE WITH MINIMAL OR NO SUPERVISION

1. Functional capacity ≥8 METs or twice the level of occupational demand
2. Appropriate hemodynamic response to exercise (increase in DP with increasing workload) and recovery
3. Appropriate ECG response at peak exercise with normal or unchanged conduction, stable or absent arrhythmias, and stable and acceptable (i.e., <1mm ST-segment depression) ischemic response
4. Cardiac symptoms stable or absent
5. Stable and/or controlled baseline HR and BP
6. Adequate management of risk factor intervention strategy and safe exercise participation such that the patient demonstrates independent and effective management of risk factors with associated positive changes in those risk factors
7. Demonstrated knowledge of the disease process, signs and symptoms, medication use and side effects
8. Demonstrated compliance and success with a program of risk intervention

ing exercise monitoring and supervision, the progression of patients from Phase II to Phase III should be based on a variety of objectives and outcomes. The shift from continuous ECG monitoring to intermittent monitoring or self-monitoring should take place independent of the decision for terminating clinical supervision. No specific guidelines are provided regarding the duration of ECG monitoring; however monitoring should be discontinued as soon as it is medically feasible. This is a decision best reached by the physician with input from the rehabilitation team. General criteria for such decisions are presented in Table 8–6.

Not all patients will be able to, or wish to, participate in a supervised program. Many choose to exercise at

TABLE 8–7. PRESCRIPTION GUIDELINES FOR HOME EXERCISE

Angina Patients	Recommended Intensity
• 0 to 1.5 mm ST-segment depression and no angina on discharge GXT	70 to 85% peak HR
• ST-segment depression ≥ 2 mm at HR > 135	70 to 85% of HR associated with onset of 1.5 mm ST-segment depression
• ST-segment depression ≥ 2 mm at HR < 135	High-risk: Suggest further medical management
• Angina with or without ST-segment depression	70 to 85% of HR at onset of angina
Other Considerations	
• Deconditioned patients (4–5 MET capacity)	60 to 75% of peak HR
• Non-cardiac limitations (PVD, COPD, orthopedic limitations)	60 to 85% of peak HR
• Initiation of β-blockers (in the absence of exercise test data)	Standard prescription based on criteria other than HR such as RPE

home based on expense, schedule flexibility, etc. Advantages to exercising under supervision include group support, professional feedback and monitoring, increased access to ergometry, and availability of emergency support. Table 8–7 provides guidelines for home exercise.

RESISTANCE TRAINING

Improving muscular strength and endurance are important complements to cardiorespiratory conditioning for cardiac rehabilitation patients. Resistance exercise may not be appropriate for some patients, including those with congestive heart failure (CHF), severe valvular disease, uncontrolled arrhythmias, or significant left ventricular dysfunction. Nevertheless, there is ample evidence to suggest that resistance exercise is safe in appropriately selected patients. Resistance training, however, should generally be deferred until 4 to 6 weeks of supervised cardiorespiratory endurance exercise have been completed. Although BP may be higher and HR lower during resistance exercise, less myocardial ischemia and fewer arrhythmias occur with resistance exercise compared with endurance exercise at a similar rate-pressure product. The reduced ischemia is presumably related to the elevated DBP associated with resistance exercise, which may enhance coronary perfusion.

Little quantitative information exists for Phase II patient resistance training. The use of elastic bands, light hand weights, and resistive tubing may be incorporated, provided that BP and continuous ECG monitoring are utilized. Exercise endpoints should be consistent with those outlined in Table 5–4 and the rate-pressure product should not exceed that during prescribed endurance exercise or that which the individual has achieved during a

TABLE 8–8. INDICATIONS FOR RESISTANCE EXERCISE
TRAINING FOR OUTPATIENTS

1. Four to six weeks after myocardial infarction or CABG
2. One to two weeks following PTCA or other revascularization
   procedure, except for CABG, without myocardial infarction
3. Four to six weeks in supervised aerobic program or completion
   of Phase II
4. Diastolic blood pressure <105 mm Hg
5. Peak exercise capacity of >5 METs
6. Not compromised by CHF, unstable symptoms, or arrhythmias

GXT. Outpatient indications for resistance exercise training are outlined in Table 8–8.

OTHER CONSIDERATIONS

Several types and manifestations of cardiac disease warrant special consideration in the development and
implementation of the exercise prescription. In all cases,
exercise prescription should be based on both objective
data from a recent symptom-limited GXT if available, as
well as subjective data regarding clinical status, response
to exercise, etc. Table 8–9 summarizes special considerations for prescription and clinical supervision of exercise. "Key factors" represent those conditions that are
particular to the specified population and to which exercise professionals should be attentive in their assessment
of those patients. Formulation of the exercise prescription in these patients should also consider different variables, as outlined in the "Exercise Prescription" section
of Table 8–9.

TABLE 8–9. SPECIAL CONSIDERATIONS FOR EARLY
REHABILITATION

Classification	Key Factors	Exercise Prescription
CABG or valvular surgery	• Incisional discomfort • Infectious processes • Anemia	• RPE of 11–14 • HR_{rest} + 30 beats/min (if HR is a desired limitation for intensity) • Range of motion for trunk and upper extremities • Muscular strength and endurance for upper extremities
PTCA (or similar procedure), MI, or angina	• Signs or symptoms of continued ischemia • Anxiety • Symptom denial • New ischemia (signs or symptoms • Resting (unstable) angina	• HR criteria if below ECG signs of ischemia • Limited by symptoms • RPE
Silent ischemia	• Associated signs (e.g., shortness-of-breath, nausea, general malaise) • Sudden decrease in exercise capacity • Sudden changes in overall condition or "sense of well-being" (prodromal symptoms)	• RPE preferred for monitoring

Continued on Next Page

TABLE 8–9. SPECIAL CONSIDERATIONS FOR EARLY
REHABILITATION *Continued*

Classification	Key Factors	Exercise Prescription
Severe LV dysfunction and CHF	• Significant weight gain (>4 lb) over short duration (1–2 days) • Decreased (or failure to increase) SBP during exercise • Resting or abnormal exercise shortness-of-breath	• RPE • SBP response to exertion • Symptoms
Pacemakers or AICDs	• Pacemaker type and method of function • Symptoms similar to pacemaker insertion • AICD threshold discharge rate • Ectopy or ventricular tachycardia	• RPE • HR (if available from post-insertion GXT) • HR and intensity threshold for exercise-induced ventricular tachycardia • Ventricular ectopy pattern(s)
Heart transplant	• Delayed and attenuated exercise HR response • Elevated resting HR • Signs of rejection • Infection • Medication side effects	• RPE • Signs and symptoms

REFERENCES

1. Guidelines for Cardiac Rehabilitation Programs. American Association of Cardiovascular and Pulmonary Rehabilitation Programs, 2nd Ed. Champaign, IL: Human Kinetic Publishers, 1994.
2. Fletcher GA, Froelicher VF, Hartley LH, Haskell WL, and Pollock ML. AHA Medical Scientific Statement. Exercise Standards—A Statement for Health Professionals from the American Heart Association. *Circulation 82*:2286–2322, 1990.
3. Health and Public Policy Committee, American College of Physicians: Cardiac Rehabilitation Services. *Ann Intern Med 15*:671–673, 1988.
4. Hillegass EA and Sadowsky HS (eds.), Essentials of Cardiopulmonary Physical Therapy. Philadelphia: WB Saunders, 1994.

chapter 9

EXERCISE PRESCRIPTION FOR PULMONARY PATIENTS

Exercise training is a key component of pulmonary rehabilitation programs. Documented benefits of exercise training in patients with respiratory disease include:[1,2]

- Increased functional capacity and/or endurance
- Increased functional status
- Decreased severity of dyspnea
- Improved quality of life

These improvements can be expected from patients regardless of the severity of pre-existing lung dysfunction. While it is true that exercise prescription should be individualized for healthy subjects and for patients with coronary artery disease, this concept is even more important for patients with pulmonary disease. At the present time there is no evidence that the principles of exercise training should be different for patients with various respiratory diseases, for example, asthma, chronic obstructive pulmonary disease (COPD), and interstitial lung disease. Although the following guidelines apply to all patients with respiratory disorders, the majority of available data has been obtained from those with COPD.

EXERCISE PRESCRIPTION

MODE OF EXERCISE

Any mode of aerobic exercise training involving large muscle groups is appropriate for pulmonary patients. Walking is strongly recommended since it is the basis of locomotion and is involved in many activities of daily living. Alternative modes of exercise include cycle ergometry and rowing. It is important that patients have activities—either primary or alternative activities—that can be performed indoors in case of inclement weather.

FREQUENCY

The recommended minimal goal for exercise frequency is 3 to 5 days per week. For some individuals, an every other day exercise schedule provides flexibility and time for recovery. Individuals with a lower functional capacity may require more frequent (e.g., daily) exercise training for optimal improvement.

INTENSITY

Intensity and duration of exercise training are closely interrelated. At present there is no consensus as to the "optimal" intensity of exercise training for pulmonary patients. At least 4 different approaches have been recommended [3-6] (Table 9–1). All or none of these strategies may work for a specific patient. The exercise professional should closely monitor initial exercise sessions and be ready to adjust intensity and/or duration according to patient responses.

In summary, there is no proven optimal intensity for exercise training in patients with respiratory disease. Rather, vastly different methods have been used with some degree of success. The exercise professional who prescribes exercise training for a patient with lung disease should select an intensity based on clinical and GXT data and a discussion with the patient as to their specific

TABLE 9–1. STRATEGIES FOR SETTING EXERCISE INTENSITY FOR PULMONARY PATIENTS

1. **Exercise at 50% of $\dot{V}o_{2peak}$**
   This intensity is consistent with the minimal intensity recommended for apparently healthy adults. Since the vast majority of patients with moderate to severe lung disease are deconditioned, training at this threshold intensity for improvement of aerobic capacity should improve exercise performance in patients with COPD. In addition, it is anticipated that adherence may be enhanced and the risk of injury reduced at this moderate exercise intensity

2. **Exercise at an intensity above the anaerobic threshold (AT)**
   The rationale for this approach is that minute ventilation (V_E) can be reduced after exercise training, provided that the training intensity is sufficient to cause metabolic acidosis. In a study of hospitalized patients with mild COPD there were significantly greater changes in exercise variables, including a reduction in V_E and lactate, in a group of patients who trained above the AT, compared to a group which trained below the AT.[3] However, it is important to recognize that many patients with severe COPD may not achieve metabolic acidosis during a GXT,[4] while others may accumulate lactate from the onset of exercise. Furthermore, any difficulty in accurately identifying the AT adds a second limitation to this strategy

Continued on Next Page

TABLE 9–1. *Continued*

3. Exercise at a near-maximal intensity

The principle of high intensity exercise training is based on the observation that patients with moderate to severe COPD can sustain ventilation at a high percentage of their maximal minute ventilatory volume (MVV). In one study,[4] 52 patients trained at an intensity of 95% of their $\dot{V}O_{2peak}$ from an initial maximal treadmill GXT. Although most individuals could only sustain this intensity for a few minutes, they significantly increased their endurance over time. As a group, the patients exhibited a significant increase in exercise time and reported less breathlessness and fatigue. Interestingly, whether or not a given patient reached AT during the initial GXT had no effect on the efficacy of the training

4. Use ratings of dyspnea to define intensity

The majority of patients with moderate to severe respiratory disease are limited by exertional dyspnea. It is therefore possible to prescribe exercise intensity based on dyspnea ratings (Figure 9–1) just as perceived exertion can be used to prescribe exercise intensity for apparently healthy individuals.[5] The target dyspnea rating is 3 (moderate) for exercise training at an intensity of 50% $\dot{V}O_{2peak}$ and 6 (between severe and very severe) for training at an intensity of 85% $\dot{V}O_{2peak}$ in this example. A preliminary study[6] demonstrated that patients with COPD can achieve a target $\dot{V}O_{2}$ within +15%, based on dyspnea ratings obtained from a previous GXT. As with RPE use, the accuracy of using the dyspnea rating scale to determine exercise intensity in patients with COPD is better at higher intensities. This approach provides a specific, easily quantified guideline for patients to self-monitor their intensity of breathlessness during routine exertional tasks. Furthermore, using dyspnea rating during exercise instills in the patient the understanding that it is appropriate and acceptable to experience some dyspnea during exercise training

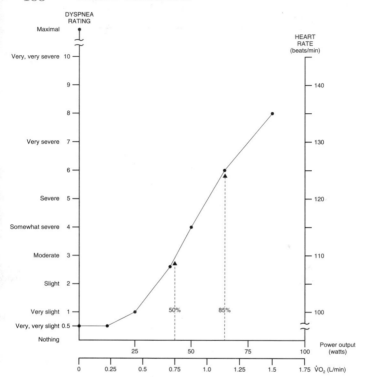

FIG. 9–1. Dyspnea ratings and heart rate responses during an incremental GXT in a patient with severe COPD. From Reference 5.

goals. Early sessions should be supervised so that either (1) appropriate adjustments can be made to the exercise intensity (or alternately, to the duration or frequency) or (2) a different strategy can be tried.

DURATION

While the minimal goal for exercise duration is 20 to 30 minutes of continuous activity, for many patients with chronic respiratory disease this duration may not be attainable at the start of an exercise training program. Therefore, some patients may only be able to exercise at a specified intensity for a few minutes because of dyspnea, leg discomfort, or other symptoms. Intermittent exercise, that is, repetitive exercise-rest periods, may be necessary for the initial training sessions until the patient can achieve sustained physical exertion.

SPECIAL CONSIDERATIONS

PURSED-LIPS BREATHING

Patients with obstructive airway disease (in particular, asthma, COPD, and cystic fibrosis) should be instructed in pursed-lips breathing during exercise. Simple patient instructions for pursed-lips breathing are:

- Breathe in through your nose
- Keep your lips firmly together except at the very center
- Breathe out twice as long as you breathe in
- When exhaling, blow the air out with a firm steady effort

The benefits of pursed-lips breathing are:

- Decreased frequency of respiration
- Increased tidal volume
- Improved oxygenation
- Provides the patient with a sense of control over breathing distress

SUPPLEMENTAL OXYGEN

As described in Chapter 4, some measure of the blood oxygenation (P_aO_2 or S_aO_2) should be made during the initial GXT. In addition, oximetry is recommended for the initial exercise training sessions in order to evaluate possible exercise-induced O_2 desaturation. Based on the recommendations of the Nocturnal Oxygen Therapy Trial,[7] supplemental O_2 is indicated for patients with:

- P_aO_2 ≤55 mmHg, or
- S_aO_2 ≤88% while breathing room air

Those same guidelines apply when considering supplemental oxygen during exercise training. The flow rate for O_2 should be titrated in order to maintain S_aO_2 >88% throughout the exercise period.

Some patients may benefit from supplemental O_2 even though these criteria are not met. A trial of oxygen versus room air may be helpful to evaluate the benefits of oxygen in patients who are extremely breathless during activities despite adequate blood oxygenation. It is still unclear whether the addition of supplemental O_2 alters the magnitude of the training effect.

ALTERNATIVE MODES OF EXERCISE TRAINING

CONTINUOUS POSITIVE AIRWAY PRESSURE (CPAP)

Dynamic hyperinflation is a physiological consequence of physical exertion in many patients with obstructive airway disease. Dynamic hyperinflation increases the elastic recoil of the lung parenchyma; the added elastic load must be overcome by the work of the respiratory muscles in order to begin inspiration. CPAP has been shown to counterbalance the added elastic recoil and thereby "unload" the respiratory muscles and reduce the sense of dyspnea.

The use of CPAP (usually at a pressure of 5 to 10 cm H_2O) can increase exercise duration and/or decrease breathlessness in patients with COPD and those with cystic fibrosis.[8,9] Therefore, a trial of CPAP may be considered in individual patients during exercise training, since it may allow patients to exercise longer with less dyspnea. CPAP can be delivered to the patient via face mask or mouthpiece and can be titrated upward from an initial level of 2 to 3 cm H_2O, increasing by 2 to 3 cm H_2O based on the patient's subjective ratings of dyspnea or breathing discomfort. Additional studies are required before CPAP can be routinely applied for exercise training purposes.

UPPER BODY RESISTANCE TRAINING

Resistance training of the upper extremities is an integral part of many pulmonary rehabilitation programs.[1,10] Typical exercises include high repetition, low intensity efforts of the arm and shoulder muscles.[10,11] These exercises can be done using manual resistance or with light weights (1 to 2 kg). Patients should be encouraged to coordinate breathing with upper extremity movement; usually expiration is linked with the motion of the arms requiring the greatest effort.

RESISTIVE INSPIRATORY MUSCLE TRAINING (RIMT)

Resistive inspiratory muscle training may be considered in conjunction with or following an exercise training program. The major indications for RIMT are:

- Patients who remain symptomatic and functionally limited despite otherwise optimal therapy
- Patients with decreased respiratory muscle strength [decreased values for inspiratory (PI_{max}) and expiratory (PE_{max}) mouth pressures]
- Absence of severe hyperinflation on chest radiograph

Various studies have demonstrated that respiratory muscle strength and endurance can be increased with RIMT. However, it is unclear whether these physiological changes contribute to consistent improvements in clinical outcome.[12] In a small number of controlled studies dyspnea has been shown to be reduced with RIMT in patients with COPD.[12,13] RIMT may be considered in an individual patient using guidelines outlined in Table 9–2. Appropriate clinical variables such as dyspnea ratings, PI_{max} and PE_{max}, and exercise performance should be measured before and after a trial of RIMT.

TABLE 9–2. GUIDELINES FOR RESISTIVE INSPIRATORY
MUSCLE TRAINING

1. Frequency	Minimum of 4 to 5 days per week
2. Intensity	25 to 35% of PI_{max} measured at functional residual capacity (FRC)
3. Duration	Two 15-minute sessions or one 30-minute session per day. If this cannot be achieved, the intensity can be reduced.

PROGRAM DESIGN AND SUPERVISION

The design and supervision of an exercise training program for patients with respiratory disease depend on multiple factors, including staff availability, facilities for testing and training, and number of patients. Inpatient exercise-based rehabilitation programs should be considered for patients who have a very limited functional status and for those with unstable disease. Inpatient exercise sessions also provide an excellent setting for instruction of both the patient and family members.

There is tremendous variability in current outpatient programs. These vary from patients participating in supervised exercise sessions 5 days per week at a clinic, hospital, or community-based rehabilitation setting to 1 supervised session per week with additional unsupervised training in the patient's home, at a public facility, or fitness center. It is essential that program design and supervision be flexible and adapted to local conditions, opportunities, and constraints.

Most formal exercise training programs for pulmonary patients last 6 to 8 weeks, with physiological and/or clinical benefits noticeable by the end of the program. Exercise prescription, especially intensity, can be modified at any time during the 6 to 8 week period. Upon completion of the program each patient should be given a written exercise prescription with clear concise instructions in order to maintain the improved status. Longer term community-based programs are beneficial in this population in encouraging continued participation. Ideally, periodic clinical follow-up with repeat testing should be scheduled to enhance the patient's compliance with his/her exercise training. However, geographical and financial factors may limit this possibility.

REFERENCES

1. American Association of Cardiovascular and Pulmonary Rehabilitation: Position paper on scientific basis of pulmonary rehabilitation. *J Cardiopulm Rehab* 10:418–441, 1990.
2. Report of the European Respiratory Society Rehabilitation and Chronic Care Scientific Group: *Pulmonary rehabilitation in chronic obstructive pulmonary disease (COPD) with recommendations for its use,* prepared by C Donner and P Howard. *Eur Respir J* 5:266–275, 1992.
3. Casaburi R, Patessio A, Ioli F, Zanaboni S, Donner CF, and Wasserman K: Reductions in exercise lactic acidosis and ventilation as a result of exercise training in patients with obstructive lung disease. *Am Rev Respir Dis* 143:9–18, 1991.
4. Punzal PA, Ries AL, Kaplan RM, and Prewitt LM: Maximum intensity exercise training in patients with chronic obstructive pulmonary disease. *Chest* 100:618–623, 1991.
5. Faryniarz K and Mahler DA: Writing an exercise prescription for patients with COPD. *J Respir Dis* 11:638–644, 1990.
6. Horowitz MB and Mahler DA: The validity of using dyspnea ratings for exercise prescription in patients with COPD. *Am Rev Respir Dis* 147(suppl.):A744, 1993.
7. Nocturnal Oxygen Therapy Trial Group. Continuous or Nocturnal Oxygen Therapy in Hypoxemic Chronic Obstructive Lung Disease: a clinical trial. *Ann Intern Med* 93:391–398, 1980.
8. Henke KG, Regnis JA, and Bye PTP: Benefits of Continuous Positive Airway Pressure during Exercise in Cystic Fibrosis

and Relationship to Disease Severity. *Am Rev Respir Dis* *148*:1272–1276, 1993.

9. O'Donnell DE, Sanii R, and Younes M: Improvement in exercise endurance in patients with chronic airflow limitation using continuous positive airway pressure. *Am Rev Respir Dis 133*:1510–1514, 1988.

10. Lake FR, Henderson K, Briffa T, Openshaw J, and Musk AW: Upper-Limb and Lower-Limb Exercise Training in Patients with Chronic Airflow Obstruction. *Chest 97*:1077–1082, 1990.

11. Simpson K, Killian K, McCartney N, Stubbing DG, and Jones NL: Randomized controlled trial of weightlifting exercise in patients with chronic airflow limitation. *Thorax 47*:70–75, 1992.

12. Smith K, Cook D, Guyatt GH, Madhavan J, and Oxman AD: Respiratory Muscle Training in Chronic Airflow Limitation: A Meta-Analysis. *Am Rev Respir Dis 145*:533–539, 1992.

13. Harver A, Mahler DA, and Daubenspeck JA: Targeted Inspiratory Muscle Training Improves Respiratory Muscle Function and Reduces Dyspnea in Patients with Chronic Obstructive Pulmonary Disease. *Ann Intern Med 111*:117–124, 1989.

chapter 10

OTHER CLINICAL CONDITIONS INFLUENCING EXERCISE PRESCRIPTION

HYPERTENSION

Over 50 million Americans are hypertensive, as defined by either a resting BP ≥140/90 mm Hg and/or current use of anti-hypertensive medication.[1] The prevalence of hypertension rises sharply with age and is higher in men than in women and in blacks compared with whites. It may be categorized as primary (cause unknown) or secondary (cause due to identifiable endocrine or structural disorders). The 1993 classification system recommended by the Joint Committee on Detection, Evaluation, and Treatment of Hypertension presented in Table 3–4 describes the stages of hypertension. Although mild hypertension is the most common form of high blood pressure in the adult population, all stages are associated with increased risk of nonfatal cardiovascular events and renal disease.

Blood pressure is determined by cardiac output and total peripheral resistance (TPR), and therefore can be elevated either as a result of elevated cardiac output, increased TPR, or both. Initial non-pharmacological treatment for hypertension includes:

- Lose weight if overweight
- Limit alcohol intake to no more than 1 ounce of ethanol per day (24 ounces of beer, 8 ounces of wine, or 2 ounces of 100 proof whiskey)
- Reduce sodium intake to less than 100 mmol per day (<2.3 grams of sodium or <6 grams of sodium chloride)
- Maintain adequate dietary potassium, calcium, and magnesium intake
- Stop smoking and reduce dietary saturated fat and cholesterol intake for overall cardiovascular health. Reducing fat intake also helps reduce caloric intake—important for control of weight and non-insulin dependent diabetes

Treatment that is refractory to this approach typically requires medications that lower either cardiac output or TPR (see Appendix A for specific antihypertensive medications and their effects on the exercise response).

ACSM makes the following recommendations regarding exercise testing and training of persons with hypertension:[2]

- Mass exercise testing is not advocated to determine those individuals at high risk for developing hypertension in the future as a result of an exaggerated exercise blood pressure response. However, if exercise test results are available and an individual has an exercise blood pressure response above the 85th percentile, this information does provide some indication of risk stratification for that patient and the necessity for appropriate lifestyle behavior counseling to ameliorate this increase

- Endurance exercise training by individuals who are at high risk for developing hypertension will reduce the rise in blood pressure that occurs with time, thus justifying its use as a nonpharmacological strategy to reduce the incidence of hypertension in susceptible individuals
- Endurance exercise training will elicit an average reduction of 10 mm Hg for both systolic and diastolic blood pressures in individuals with mild essential hypertension (blood pressures in the range of 140 to 180/90 to 105 mm Hg) and even greater reductions in blood pressure in patients with secondary hypertension due to renal dysfunction
- The recommended mode, frequency, duration, and intensity of exercise are generally the same as those for apparently healthy individuals. Exercise training at somewhat lower intensities (e.g., 40 to 70% $\dot{V}O_{2max}$) appears to lower blood pressure as much, or more, than exercise at higher intensities, which may be especially important in specific hypertensive populations, such as the elderly
- Based on the high number of exercise-related health benefits and low risk for morbidity/mortality, it seems reasonable to recommend exercise as part of the initial treatment strategy for individuals with mild to moderate essential hypertension
- Individuals with marked elevations in blood pressure should add endurance exercise training to their treatment regimen only after initiating pharmacologic therapy; exercise may reduce their blood pressure further, allow them to decrease their antihypertensive medications, and attenuate their risk for premature mortality
- Resistance training is not recommended as the primary form of exercise training for hypertensive individuals. With the exception of circuit weight training, resistance training has not consistently been shown to lower blood pressure. Thus resistance training is recommended as a component of a well-rounded fitness program, but not when done independently

See Table 10–1 for additional exercise and prescription guidelines.

PERIPHERAL VASCULAR DISEASE

Peripheral vascular disease (PVD) is a generic term, and includes vascular insufficiencies such as arteriosclerosis, arterial stenosis, Raynaud's phenomenon (an abnormal vasomotor tone exacerbated by cold exposure), and Buerger's disease (an inflammation of the sheath encapsulating the neurovascular bundle in the extremities). Peripheral arteriosclerosis is common in the elderly, and is often associated with hypertension and hyperlipidemia. PVD is frequently observed in patients with CAD and cerebrovascular disease, and may also be seen in patients with diabetes mellitus.

Patients with PVD experience ischemic pain (claudication) during physical activity as a result of a mismatch between active muscle oxygen supply and demand. The various manifestations of the symptoms may be described as burning, searing, aching, tightness, or cramping. The pain is most often experienced in the calf of the leg but can begin in the buttock region and radiate down the leg. The symptoms typically disappear upon cessation of exercise.

Assessment of the extent of disease is possible through many procedures, including physical examination, Doppler studies, ankle-to-arm pressure indices, nuclear medicine flow studies, and arteriography. Severe occlusive disease is treated initially with exercise and medications that decrease blood viscosity. Treatment with angioplasty or bypass grafting may also be indicated. Weight-bearing exercise is preferred to facilitate greater functional changes but may not be well-tolerated initially. As such, prescription of non-weightbearing exercise (which may permit a greater intensity or longer duration)

TABLE 10-1. RECOMMENDATIONS FOR SPECIAL POPULATIONS

	Exercise Test Methods	Exercise Prescription	Exercise Precautions
Hypertension	Standard methods and protocols LVH may interfere with ECG interpretation; therefore thallium testing may be preferred for diagnostic testing	Frequency: 4–5/week Duration: 30–60 min Intensity: 40–70% $\dot{V}O_{2max}$ High intensity and isometric activities should be avoided Weight training should involve low resistance with high reps	Meds may decrease TPR: longer cool-down Meds limiting cardiac output: use RPE as an adjunct to HR Diuretics may cause a decrease in K^+, leading to arrhythmias Avoid Valsalva maneuvers
Peripheral Vascular Disease	Multi-stage discontinuous protocol may be necessary to achieve peak O_2 consumption Use scale for subjective ratings of pain If severe, GXT using arm ergometry may be necessary	Weightbearing activities are preferred, but non-weightbearing activities may allow longer duration and higher intensity exercise Daily exercise to maximum tolerable pain with intermittent rest periods	

Continued on Following Two Pages

TABLE 10-1. Continued

	Exercise Test Methods	Exercise Prescription	Exercise Precautions
		Frequency/duration: begin with 20 min, twice daily (or less), with a goal of increasing to one 40–60 min session	
Diabetes	May require modification of standard protocols or arm ergometry Autonomic neuropathy may prevent achievement of age-predicted HR_{max}	Daily exercise for IDDM Duration of 20–30 min/session to achieve glucose control NIDDM: maximize caloric expenditure if obese May need to use RPE as adjunct to HR for monitoring exercise intensity	Especially when beginning a program, monitor blood glucose before and after exercise Adjustments in carbohydrate intake and/or insulin may be needed Exercise caution when exercising in hot weather

Continued on Next Page

TABLE 10–1. *Continued*

	Exercise Test Methods	Exercise Prescription	Exercise Precautions
Obesity	Low level treadmill testing Use of cycle or arm ergometry may enhance testing capability	Goal: increase caloric expenditure First choice: walking Alternative modes: stairclimbing, cycling, water exercise Intensity at low end of target heart rate range Duration sufficient to cause expenditure of 200–300 kcal/session	Avoid stress on joints Choose setting that minimizes social stigmata Monitor muscle soreness and orthopedic problems

is a suitable alternative. See Table 10–1 for exercise testing and prescription guidelines. A subjective grading scale for PVD pain is shown below:

•	Grade I	Definite discomfort or pain, but only of initial or modest levels (established, but minimal)
•	Grade II	Moderate discomfort or pain from which the patient's attention can be diverted, for example by conversation
•	Grade III	Intense pain (short of Grade IV) from which the patient's attention cannot be diverted
•	Grade IV	Excruciating and unbearable pain

As functional capacity improves with less peripheral limitation, central cardiac limitations may assume greater importance. This may require modification of the program in terms of supervision, intensity, and duration.

DIABETES MELLITUS

Diabetes mellitus is a disease associated with problems in controlling blood glucose, resulting primarily in hyperglycemia. There are two major types of diabetes mellitus. Insulin-dependent diabetes mellitus (IDDM—also referred to as Type I or juvenile-onset diabetes) results from a pancreatic deficiency in insulin production or related metabolic abnormalities. Non-insulin dependent diabetes mellitus (NIDDM—also called Type II or maturity-onset diabetes) is usually associated with decreased cellular insulin sensitivity. IDDM diabetics are often dependent on regular injections of insulin, usually given twice daily or through an infusion pump. NIDDM diabetics may benefit from oral hypoglycemic agents rather than injections of insulin, although exogenous insulin is sometimes used. Since insulin facilitates the cellular absorption of glucose, a lack of sufficient circulating insulin usually results in hyperglycemia.

The response to exercise in the IDDM diabetic depends upon a variety of factors, including the adequacy of control by exogenous insulin. If the diabetic is under appropriate control or only slightly hyperglycemic without ketosis, exercise decreases blood glucose concentration and a lower insulin dosage may be required. However, problems can arise during exercise if the diabetic is not under adequate control. A lack of sufficient insulin prior to exercise may impair glucose transport into the muscles limiting the availability of glucose as an energy substrate. To compensate, use of free fatty acids increases and ketone bodies are produced, possibly leading to the development of ketosis. In addition, the resulting greater glucose production further exacerbates the hyperglycemic state. For these reasons, IDDM diabetics must be under adequate control prior to beginning an exercise program. Serum glucose concentrations in the general range of 200 to 400 mg% (mg/dL) require medical supervision during exercise, while exercise is contraindicated for those with fasting serum values >400 mg% pending medical follow-up.

On the other hand, because exercise has an insulin-like effect, exercise-induced hypoglycemia is the most common problem experienced by exercising diabetics. Hypoglycemia may result when too much insulin is present, or if there is accelerated absorption of insulin from the injection site, both of which may occur with exercise. Hypoglycemia can not only occur during exercise, but may occur up to 4 to 6 hours following an exercise bout. To counteract this response, the diabetic may need to reduce his/her insulin dosage or increase carbohydrate intake prior to exercising.

The risk of hypoglycemic events may be minimized by taking the following precautions:

- Monitor blood glucose frequently when initiating an exercise program
- Decrease insulin dose (by 1 to 2 units as prescribed by the physician) or increase carbohydrate (CHO) intake (10 to 15 g CHO per 30 minutes of exercise) prior to an exercise bout
- Inject insulin in an area such as the abdomen that is not active during exercise
- Avoid exercise during periods of peak insulin activity
- Eat carbohydrate snacks before and during prolonged exercise bouts
- Be knowledgeable of the signs and symptoms of hypo- and hyperglycemia
- Exercise with a partner

Other precautions that must be taken include (1) proper footwear and practice of good foot hygiene, (2) awareness that β-blockers and other medications may interfere with the ability to discern hypoglycemic symptoms and/or angina, and (3) awareness that exercise in excessive heat may cause problems in diabetics with peripheral neuropathy. Patients with advanced retinopathy should not perform activities which cause excessive jarring or marked increases in blood pressure. Patients should have physician approval to resume exercise training following laser treatment. See Table 10–1 for exercise testing and prescription guidelines.

OBESITY

Obesity may be functionally defined as the percent body fat at which disease risk increases. Body fat is reduced when a chronic negative caloric balance exists. It is recommended that both an increase in caloric expenditure through exercise and a decrease in caloric intake be used to accomplish this goal. Exercise increases energy expenditure and slows the rate of fat-free tissue loss that occurs when a person loses weight by severe caloric restriction. Exercise also helps maintain the resting metabolic rate and thus the rate of weight loss.

Obese individuals are invariably sedentary and many have had poor experiences with exercise in the past. The exercise professional should interview the obese participant to determine past exercise history, potential scheduling difficulties, and the locations where exercise might be performed (e.g., sports club, home, street, school gym or track, etc.). This may increase adherence to an agreed upon exercise program. See Table 10–1 for exercise testing and prescription guidelines.

The initial exercise prescription should be based on low intensity and progressively longer durations of activity. On the basis of each person's response to the initial exercise program, the exercise professional should eventually work toward increasing the intensity to bring the person into a target heart rate range suitable for cardiorespiratory conditioning. The higher intensity will allow for a shorter duration per session, or fewer sessions per week for the same weekly energy expenditure. In addition, the transition to higher intensity exercise will increase the number of opportunities to incorporate activities that naturally require a higher rate of energy expenditure. However, for many (especially older) obese subjects, a walking or other low intensity exercise program may be all they desire, and movement toward a more intense program may not be warranted. The needs and goals of the obese subject must be individually matched with the proper exercise program to achieve long-term weight management.

PROGRAMS FOR REDUCING BODY FATNESS

An excessive percentage of body fat is associated with increased risk for development of hypertension, diabetes, CAD, and other chronic diseases. Recent evidence indicates that "central obesity" (fat deposited primarily in the trunk or abdominal region) is particularly problematic. In addition, obesity often carries a negative social stigma and is associated with a reduced physical working capacity. Since reduction of body fatness is a need or a goal of many exercise program participants, exercise prescriptions should be designed to aid in accomplishing this objective. This section presents the principles that should be employed in modifying body composition.

CALORIC BALANCE

Body composition is determined by a complex set of genetic and behavioral factors. Though the contributing variables are many, the fundamental determinant of body weight and body composition is caloric balance. Caloric balance refers to the difference between caloric intake (the energy equivalent of the food ingested) and caloric expenditure (the energy equivalent of resting metabolic rate, activity, thermic effect of food, etc.). The First Law of Thermodynamics states that energy is neither created nor destroyed; therefore, body weight is lost when caloric expenditure exceeds caloric intake (negative balance) and weight is gained when the opposite situation exists. One pound of fat is equivalent to approximately 3500 kcal of energy (1 kg ≈ 7700 kcal). Although it is predictable that shifts in caloric balance will be accompanied by changes in body weight, the nature of the weight change varies markedly with the specific behaviors that lead to the caloric imbalance. For example, fasting and extreme caloric restriction (starvation and semistarvation diets) cause substantial losses of water and fat-free tissue. In contrast, an exercise-induced negative caloric balance results in weight loss consisting primarily of fat. High resistance exercise programs may lead to a gain in fat-free weight, while cardiorespiratory endurance training usually results in a maintenance of (or slight increase in) fat-free weight. Both types of programs can contribute to a loss of body fat, although aerobic activity is more efficient because it involves a sustained, high rate of energy expenditure.

RECOMMENDED WEIGHT LOSS PROGRAMS

For most persons, the optimal approach to weight loss combines a mild caloric restriction with regular endurance exercise and avoids nutritional deficiencies. A desirable weight loss program is one that meets the following criteria:

- Provides intake not lower than 1200 kcal/day for normal adults and ensures a proper blend of foods to meet nutritional requirements. (Note: this requirement may not be appropriate for children, older individuals, and athletes)
- Includes foods acceptable to the dieter in terms of sociocultural background, usual habits, taste, costs, and ease in acquisition and preparation
- Provides a negative caloric balance (not to exceed 500 to 1000 kcal/day), resulting in gradual weight loss without metabolic derangements, such as ketosis
- Results in a maximal weight loss of 1 kg/week

- Includes the use of behavior modification techniques to identify and eliminate diet habits that contribute to malnutrition
- Includes an exercise program that promotes a daily caloric expenditure of 300 or more kcal. For many participants, this may be best accomplished with low intensity, long duration exercise, such as walking
- Provides that new eating and physical activity habits can be continued for life in order to maintain the achieved lower body weight

In designing the exercise component of a weight loss program, the balance between intensity and duration of exercise should be manipulated to promote a high total caloric expenditure (300 to 500 kcal per session and 1000 to 2000 kcal per week for adults). Obese individuals are at an increased relative risk for orthopedic injury, and this may require that the intensity of exercise be maintained at or below the intensity recommended for improvement of cardiorespiratory endurance. Non-weightbearing activities (and/or rotation of exercise modalities) may be necessary and frequent modifications in frequency and duration may also be required.

REFERENCES

1. The Fifth Report of the Joint National Committee on Detection, Evaluation, and Treatment of High Blood Pressure (JNC V). *Arch Int Med 153*:154–183, 1993.
2. American College of Sports Medicine. Physical activity, physical fitness, and hypertension. Position Stand. *Med Sci Sports Exerc 25*:i–x, 1993.

11 ▬▬▬▬▬

EXERCISE TESTING AND PRESCRIPTION FOR CHILDREN, THE ELDERLY, AND PREGNANCY

This chapter addresses recommended procedures for exercise testing and prescription in three non-diseased special populations—children, the elderly, and pregnant women. Each of these groups possesses unique physical, physiological, and behavioral characteristics which require that special considerations be applied in exercise testing and training.

CHILDREN

EXERCISE TESTING

Fitness Testing. Measurement of physical fitness in children is a common practice in school-based physical education programs. Such testing has also been employed in public health surveys,[1,2] recreational programs, and clinical settings. Traditionally, fitness testing of children has emphasized measurement of skill-related fitness components such as agility and balance. Only recently has there been an awareness of the need to assess health-related fitness in children, a concept strongly endorsed by ACSM. Youth fitness tests should emphasize health-related measures, and criterion-referenced standards should be applied in interpreting the results of such tests.[3] Table 11-1 provides a list of field tests of physical fitness currently in wide use.[1-8]

Clinical Exercise Testing. In recent years, emphasis has been placed on the value of exercise testing to assess cardiopulmonary function and assist in the diagnosis of cardiovascular and pulmonary disease for the pediatric pop-

TABLE 11-1. REFERENCED LIST OF FIELD FITNESS TESTS FOR CHILDREN*

Fitness Component and Tests	References
Cardiorespiratory Endurance	
• Mile run/walk for time	1, 2, 4-7
• One-half mile run/walk (ages 6 to 7)	2
• Steady state jog	8
Body Composition	
• Skinfold measurements	1-4, 6
• Body Mass Index	1, 2, 4, 6
Muscular Strength/Endurance	
• Pull-ups	1, 4, 6
• Flexed arm hang	5-7
• Bent-knee sit-ups or curl-ups	1-8
• Push-ups	5
Flexibility	
• Sit-and-Reach test	1, 2, 4, 6, 8
• V-Sit Reach	5, 7

*For detailed descriptions of specific test items, the reader is referred to the references cited.

ulation. The indications for, and value of, pediatric exercise testing are essentially the same as those of an adult population. While there are many clinical uses of exercise testing in children, specific methodological concerns exist. For example, with repeated testing, it is difficult to determine whether measured changes in function are due to the implementation of an intervention program or to the normal growth and development of the child.

Additional considerations exist when testing children. Issues such as pediatric contraindications to testing, selection of test modality and appropriate protocol are all highly dependent on the physical characteristics, health status, and motivation level of the child. AHA contraindications to exercise testing in children include[9]:

- Acute inflammatory cardiac disease
- Uncontrolled congestive heart failure
- Acute myocardial infarction
- Acute pulmonary disease
- Severe systemic hypertension
- Acute renal disease
- Acute hepatitis
- Drug overdose affecting cardiorespiratory response to exercise

---

Exercise testing of children may be performed on either a treadmill or cycle ergometer. Often the physical abilities or disabilities of the child will dictate the modality to be used. Two disadvantages of cycle ergometry for children are (1) cycle ergometry requires a greater attention span than treadmill walking since the activity is self-driven, and (2) children may have underdeveloped knee extensor muscle mass. Good test protocols exist for both the treadmill and the cycle ergometer, but the chosen protocol must be flexible enough to adapt to the child's age, fitness level, and physical stature. In treadmill testing of children it is optimal to adjust grade only while leaving speed constant. This allows the child easier adaptation to stage changes. The Modified Balke protocol meets this need and is adjustable for varying age and fitness levels.

Cycle ergometers must usually be modified to fit children. Seat height, handlebar height, and pedal crank position must all be evaluated and adjusted when necessary. Most children age 8 years and older (or ≥ 125 cm or 50 in tall) can be tested on a standard cycle ergometer. The McMaster Cycle Test has been extensively used to measure $\dot{V}O_{2max}$ in children. This protocol is based on the height of the child and total exercise time is optimally only 8 to 12 minutes. Both of these protocols are shown in Table 11–2.

TABLE 11–2. PROTOCOLS SUITABLE FOR GRADED EXERCISE TESTING OF CHILDREN

Modified Balke Treadmill Protocol

Subject	Speed (mph)	Initial Grade (%)	Increment (%)	Stage Duration(min)
Poorly fit	3.00	6	2	2
Sedentary	3.25	6	2	2
Active	5.00	0	2.5	2
Athlete	5.25	0	2.5	2

The McMaster Cycle Test

Height (cm)	Initial Load (Watts)	Increments (Watts)	Step Duration (min)
<120	12.5	12.5	2
120–139.9	12.5	25	2
140–159.9	25	25	2
≥160	25	50 (boys) 25 (girls)	2

In children, it is often necessary to terminate the test prior to the attainment of maximal aerobic capacity for various reasons. In such cases, the workload should be gradually decreased and the child should be allowed to recover for at least 5 minutes by walking slowly or pedaling with no resistance. Once the child is within 20% of his or her baseline HR and BP, exercise may stop. Specific test termination criteria are similar to those for an adult (Table 5–4).

EXERCISE PRESCRIPTION

As a general rule, children tend to be more habitually active than adults and accordingly maintain adequate levels of physical fitness. Nonetheless, healthy children should be encouraged to engage in physical activity on a regular basis.[3] However, because children are anatomically, physiologically, and psychologically immature, special precautions should be applied when designing exercise programs.

Exercise safety for children should always be of primary concern. While physical activity should be strongly promoted among children, detrimental effects such as overuse syndromes or sports injuries will occur if appropriate precautions are not taken. Children may experience a higher incidence of overuse injuries or damage the epiphyseal growth plates if endurance exercise is excessive. The risk of injury can be significantly decreased by ensuring appropriate matching of competition in terms of size, maturation or skill level, use of properly fitted protective equipment, liberal adaptation of rules, and proper conditioning and skill development. Another concern in exercising children is their relative inability to adapt to thermal stress. Thermoregulation in children during heat exposure is less efficient due to a higher threshold for sweating and a lower output of the heat-activated sweat glands. Although children have a high surface area-to-body mass ratio, the efficiency of heat loss through conduction, radiation, and convection may be impaired due to a lower skin blood flow. Thus, children may be more prone to heat injury than adults. In addition, the high surface area-to-body mass ratio of children results in accelerated heat loss during exposure to cold, which increases their risk of hypothermia.

Available evidence suggests that children can safely participate in properly designed *resistance* training programs.[10] The following guidelines and principles are offered as suggestions to the individual interested in developing a sound strength training program for adolescents:

- No matter how big, strong, or mature a young man or woman appears, remember that he/she is physiologically immature
- Teach proper training techniques for all of the exercise movements involved in the program and proper breathing techniques (i.e., no breath-holding)
- Stress that exercises should be performed in a manner in which the speed is controlled avoiding ballistic (fast and jerky) movements
- Under no circumstances should a weight be used that allows less than eight repetitions to be completed per set, since heavy weights can be potentially dangerous and damaging to the developing skeletal and joint structures. It is *not* recommended that resistance exercise be performed to the point of momentary muscular fatigue
- As a training effect occurs, achieve an overload initially by increasing the number of repetitions, and then by increasing the absolute resistance
- Perform one to two sets of eight to ten different exercises (with 8 to 12 reps per set), ensuring that all of the major muscle groups are included

- Limit strength training sessions to twice per week and encourage children and adolescents to seek other forms of physical activity
- Perform full range, multi-joint exercises (as opposed to single joint exercises)
- Do not overload the skeletal and joint structures of adolescents with maximal weights
- Finally and perhaps most important, all strength-training activities should be closely supervised and monitored by appropriately trained personnel

Children with certain illnesses and physical challenges merit special attention. Such children tend to be far less active than their healthy counterparts. As a result, these children may require special adjustments in their exercise prescriptions[11] (see Table 11–3).

TABLE 11–3. EXERCISE PRESCRIPTION IN THE MANAGEMENT OF SPECIFIC PEDIATRIC DISEASES*

Disease	Purposes of Program	Recommended Activities
Anorexia nervosa	Means for behavioral modification; educate regarding lean body mass versus fat	Various; emphasize those with low energy demand
Bronchial asthma	Conditioning; possible reduction of exercise-induced bronchospasm; instill confidence	Aquatic, intermittent, long warm-up
Cerebral palsy	Increase maximal aerobic power, range of motion, ambulation; control of body mass	Depends on residual ability

Continued on Next Page

TABLE 11–3. *Continued*

Disease	Purposes of Program	Recommended Activities
Cystic fibrosis	Improve mucus clearance, training of respiratory muscles	Jogging, swimming
Diabetes mellitus	Help in metabolic control; control of body mass	Various; attempt equal daily energy output
Hemophilia	Prevent muscle atrophy and possible bleeding in joints	Swimming, cycling; avoid contact sports
Mental retardation	Socialization; increase self-esteem; prevent detraining	Recreational, intermittent, large variety
Muscular dystrophies	Increase muscle strength and endurance; prolong ambulatory phase	Swimming, calisthenics, wheelchair sports
Neurocirculatory disease	Increase effort tolerance; improve orthostatic response	Various; emphasize endurance-type activities
Obesity	Reduction of body mass and fat; conditioning; socialization and improved self-esteem	High in caloric expenditure but feasible to child; swimming
Rheumatoid arthritis	Prevent contractures and muscle atrophy; increase daily function	Swimming, calisthenics, cycling, sailing
Spina bifida	Strengthen upper body; control of body mass and fat; increase maximal aerobic power	Arm-shoulder resistance training, wheelchair sports (including endurance)

*Reprinted with permission from Reference 11.

THE ELDERLY

EXERCISE TESTING

The rationale for exercise testing within an elderly population is similar to that of any adult population. Several key points deserve mention. First, knowledge of the effects of the aging process on variables measured during exercise testing is critical to the safe and effective performance of exercise testing in the elderly. A list of such changes includes:

Resting heart rate	Little or no change
Maximal heart rate	Decreases
Maximal cardiac output	Decreases
Resting & exercise BP	Increases
Maximal oxygen uptake	Decreases
Residual volume	Increases
Vital capacity	Decreases
Reaction time	Increases
Muscular strength	Decreases
Bone mass	Decreases
Flexibility	Decreases
Fat-free body mass	Decreases
Percent body fat	Increases
Glucose tolerance	Decreases
Recovery time	Increases

Second, physiological aging does not occur uniformly across the population; therefore it is not wise to define "elderly" by any specific chronological age or set of ages. Individuals of the same age can and will differ drastically in their physiological status and response to an exercise stimulus. Third, it is difficult to distinguish effects due to deconditioning, age-related decline, and disease. Fourth, while aging is inevitable, both the pace and potential reversibility of this process may be amenable to intervention. And finally, the possibility that an active or latent disease process may be present in the subject must always be considered. In accordance with Table 2–7, medical clearance is advised prior to maximal exercise testing or their participation in vigorous exercise.

Various test protocols utilizing a variety of modalities have been used for testing the elderly population, either in their standard form or with slight modifications. In addition, many protocols have been developed for those who are highly deconditioned or physically limited. As aging increases the adaptation time to a given workload and $\dot{V}O_{2max}$ declines with age, an optimal protocol combines a prolonged warm-up and adaptation period with a low initial exercise intensity. However, no ideal protocol exists for all older adults. Other factors to be considered when selecting an exercise testing protocol for older adults[12] are presented in Table 11–4.

No specific exercise test termination criteria are necessary for the elderly population beyond those previously presented (Table 5–4). On the other hand, probable attainment of a lower $\dot{V}O_{2max}$ coupled with the increased prevalence of cardiovascular, metabolic, and orthopedic problems in the elderly leads to the reality that the test may often be terminated (either volitionally or due to achievement of established criteria) earlier than with the young adult population.

EXERCISE PRESCRIPTION

The general principles of exercise prescription (Chapter 7) apply to individuals of all ages. However, the wide range of health and fitness levels observed among older adults make generic exercise prescription more difficult.

TABLE 11-4. FACTORS TO CONSIDER WHEN SELECTING AN EXERCISE TESTING PROTOCOL FOR OLDER ADULTS*

Characteristic	Suggested Test Modification
Low $\dot{V}O_{2max}$	Start at low intensity (2–3 METs)
More time to attain a steady state	Long warm-up (>3 min), small increments in work rate (0.5–1.0 MET per stage), longer stages
Increased fatigability	Reduce total test time (ideally 8–12 min)
Increased need to monitor ECG, BP, and HR	Cycle ergometer preferred
Poor balance	Cycle ergometer preferred
Poor ambulatory ability	Increase treadmill grade rather than speed
Poor neuromuscular coordination	Increase amount of practice, may require more than one test

*Reprinted with permission from Reference 12.

Care must be taken in establishing the type, intensity, duration, and frequency of exercise:

Mode
- The exercise modality should be one that does not impose significant orthopedic stress
- The activity should be accessible, convenient, and enjoyable to the participant—all factors directly related to exercise adherence
- Consider walking, stationary cycling, water exercise, swimming, or machine-based stair climbing

Intensity
- Intensity must be sufficient to stress (overload) the cardiovascular, pulmonary, and musculoskeletal systems without overtaxing them

- High variability exists for maximal heart rates in persons over 65 years of age; thus, it is always better to use a measured maximal heart rate (HR_{max}) rather than age-predicted HR_{max} whenever possible
- For similar reasons, the HR reserve method is recommended for establishing a training HR in older individuals, rather than a straight percentage of HR_{max}
- The recommended intensity for older adults is 50 to 70% of HR reserve
- Since many older persons suffer from a variety of medical conditions, a conservative approach to prescribing aerobic exercise is initially warranted

Duration
- During the initial stages of an exercise program, some older adults may have difficulty sustaining aerobic exercise for 20 minutes; one viable option may be to perform the exercise in several 10-minute bouts throughout the day
- To avoid injury and ensure safety, older individuals should initially increase exercise duration rather than intensity

Frequency
- Alternate between days that involve primarily weightbearing and non-weightbearing exercise

Resistance Training. Recent research findings suggest that improved muscular fitness (muscular strength and muscular endurance) offers considerable benefits to older adults.[13] Resistance training may enable elderly individuals to perform activities of daily living with greater ease and counteract muscle weakness and frailty in very old persons. Some minimal level of muscular fitness is critical for individuals to retain their independence. It is believed that resistance training provides significant musculoskeletal benefits for men and women of all ages, and an appropriate level of muscular fitness is integral to ensuring that individuals are able to spend their latter years in a self-sufficient, dignified manner.

Similar to cardiorespiratory fitness, individualization of the resistance training prescription is essential and should be based on the health/fitness status and specific goals of the participant. Some guidelines follow, with reference to the intensity, frequency, and duration of exercise:

Intensity
- Perform one set of 8 to 10 exercises that train all the major muscle groups (e.g., gluteals, quadriceps, hamstrings, pectorals, latissimus dorsi, deltoids, and abdominals). Each set should involve 8 to 12 repetitions that elicit a perceived exertion rating of 12 to 13 (somewhat hard)

Frequency
- Resistance training should be performed at least twice a week, with at least 48 hours of rest between sessions

Duration
- Sessions lasting longer than 60 minutes may have a detrimental effect on exercise adherence. Adherence to the guidelines set forth in this chapter should permit individuals to complete total body resistance training sessions within 20 to 30 minutes

---

Regardless of which specific protocol is adopted, several common sense guidelines pertaining to resistance training for older adults should be followed:

- The major goal of the resistance training program is to develop sufficient muscular fitness to enhance an individual's ability to live a physically independent lifestyle

- The first several resistance training sessions should be closely supervised and monitored by trained personnel who are sensitive to the special needs and capabilities of the elderly
- Begin (the first eight weeks) with minimal resistance to allow for adaptations of the connective tissue elements
- Teach proper training techniques for all of the exercises to be used in the program
- Instruct older participants to maintain their normal breathing pattern while exercising
- As a training effect occurs, achieve an overload initially by increasing the number of repetitions, and then by increasing the resistance
- Never use a resistance that is so heavy that the exerciser cannot perform at least eight repetitions
- Stress that all exercises should be performed in a manner in which the speed is controlled (no ballistic movements should be allowed)
- Perform the exercises in a range of motion that is within a "painfree arc" (i.e., the maximum range of motion that does not elicit pain or discomfort)
- Perform multi-joint exercises (as opposed to single-joint exercises)
- Given a choice, use machines to resistance train, as opposed to free weights (machines require less skill to use, protect the back by stabilizing the user's body position, and allow the user to start with lower resistances, to increase by smaller increments, and to more easily control the exercise range of motion)
- Don't overtrain. Two strength training sessions per week are the minimum number required to produce positive physiological adaptations; depending on the circumstances, more sessions may be neither desirable nor productive
- Never permit arthritic participants to participate in strength training exercises during active periods of pain or inflammation
- Engage in a year-round resistance training program on a regular basis
- When returning from a lay-off, start with resistances ≤50% of the intensity at which they had been previously training, then gradually increase the resistance

Flexibility. An adequate range of motion in all of the joints of the body is important to maintaining an acceptable level of musculoskeletal function in older adults. Unfortunately, efforts to identify the most effective protocol for developing flexibility have been limited in comparison to the other basic components of physical fitness. What is almost universally accepted, although not documented, is the fact that maintaining adequate levels of flexibility will enhance an individual's functional capabilities (e.g., bending and twisting) and reduce injury potential (e.g., risk of muscle strains and low back problems)—particularly for the aged. A well-rounded program of stretching can counteract the usual decline in flexibility of the elderly. Not surprisingly, it is critical that a sound stretching program be included as part of each exercise session for older adults:

Intensity
- Exercises should incorporate slow movement, followed by a static stretch that is sustained for 10 to 30 seconds
- Exercises should be prescribed for every major joint (hip, back, shoulder, knee, upper trunk, and neck regions) in the body
- Three to five repetitions of each exercise should be performed
- The degree of stretch achieved should not cause pain, but rather mild discomfort

Frequency
- Stretching exercises should be performed at least three times a week (preferably daily) and should be included as an integral part of the warm-up and cool-down exercises
- Devoting an entire exercise session to flexibility may be particularly appropriate for deconditioned older adults who are beginning an exercise program

Duration
- The stretching phase of an exercise session should last approximately 15 to 30 minutes

Several guidelines pertaining to stretching by older adults should be followed:

- Always precede stretching exercises with some type of warm-up activity to increase circulation and internal body temperature
- Stretch smoothly and never bounce
- Do not stretch a joint beyond its pain-free range of motion
- Gradually ease into a stretch, and hold it only as long as it feels comfortable (10 to 30 sec)

PREGNANCY

Pregnant women represent a unique clientele because of the possible competition between exercising maternal muscle and the fetus for blood flow, oxygen delivery, glucose availability, and heat dissipation. Also, metabolic and cardiorespiratory adaptations to pregnancy may alter the responses to acute exercise and the adaptations that result from exercise training. Benefits of a properly designed prenatal exercise program include: improved aerobic and muscular fitness, facilitation of recovery from labor, enhanced maternal psychological well-being, and establishment of permanent healthy lifestyle habits.

There are no data in humans to indicate that pregnant women should limit exercise intensity and lower target heart rates because of potential adverse effects. For women who do not have any additional risk factors for adverse maternal or perinatal outcomes, the American College of Obstetricians and Gynecologists (ACOG) has established guidelines for the safe prescription of exercise[14] (see Table 11–5).

Although some pregnant women have undergone maximal exercise testing, it is not recommended in nonclinical

TABLE 11–5. AMERICAN COLLEGE OF OBSTETRICIANS AND GYNECOLOGISTS (ACOG) RECOMMENDATIONS FOR EXERCISE IN PREGNANCY AND POSTPARTUM*

1. During pregnancy, women can continue to exercise and derive health benefits even from mild to moderate exercise routines. Regular exercise (at least 3 times per week) is preferable to intermittent activity

2. Women should avoid exercise in the supine position after the first trimester. Such a position is associated with decreased cardiac output in most pregnant women. Because the remaining cardiac output will be preferentially distributed away from splanchnic beds (including the uterus) during vigorous exercise, such regimens are best avoided during pregnancy. Prolonged periods of motionless standing should also be avoided

3. Women should be aware of the decreased oxygen available for aerobic exercise during pregnancy. They should be encouraged to modify the intensity of their exercise according to maternal symptoms. Pregnant women should stop exercising when fatigued and not exercise to exhaustion. Weightbearing exercises may under some circumstances be continued at intensities similar to those prior to pregnancy throughout pregnancy. Non-weightbearing exercises, such as cycling or swimming, will minimize the risk of injury and facilitate the continuation of exercise during pregnancy

4. Morphologic changes in pregnancy should serve as a relative contraindication to types of exercise in which loss of balance could be detrimental to maternal or fetal well-being, especially in the third trimester. Further, any type of exercise involving the potential for even mild abdominal trauma should be avoided

5. Pregnancy requires an additional 300 kcal/day in order to maintain metabolic homeostasis. Thus, women who exercise during pregnancy should be particularly careful to ensure an adequate diet

6. Pregnant women who exercise in the first trimester should augment heat dissipation by ensuring adequate hydration, appropriate clothing, and optimal environmental surroundings during exercise

7. Many of the physiological and morphological changes of pregnancy persist four to six weeks postpartum. Thus, prepregnancy exercise routines should be resumed gradually based upon a woman's physical capability

*Reprinted with permission from Reference 14.

settings. Women who are appropriately screened prior to initiating exercise and who are educated regarding signs and/or symptoms for discontinuing exercise typically do not experience problems (see Table 11–6).[15] Contraindications for exercise during pregnancy have also been established by the ACOG and are listed in Table 11–7. While exercise may not be appropriate for every pregnant woman, for most pregnant women, exercise—with physician authorization—can contribute to better maternal health and offers minimal risk to the developing fetus.

Older guidelines limited maternal HR to 140 beats/min, yet, no adverse maternal or fetal effects were reported as a result of a higher training HR. The revised ACOG guidelines recommend eliminating HR and utilizing RPE as the

TABLE 11–6. REASONS TO DISCONTINUE EXERCISE AND SEEK MEDICAL ADVICE DURING PREGNANCY*†

1. Any signs of bloody discharge from the vagina
2. Any "gush" of fluid from the vagina (premature rupture of membranes)
3. Sudden swelling of the ankles, hands, or face
4. Persistent, severe headaches and/or visual disturbance; unexplained spell of faintness or dizziness
5. Swelling, pain, and redness in the calf of one leg (phlebitis)
6. Elevation of pulse rate or blood pressure that persists after exercise
7. Excessive fatigue, palpitations, chest pain
8. Persistant contractions (>6 to 8/hour) that may suggest onset of premature labor
9. Unexplained abdominal pain
10. Insufficient weight gain (<1.0 kg/month during last two trimesters)

*Participants and the exercise instructor should know these signs and symptoms, and the participant should consult the physician monitoring her pregnancy if any are encountered. Women who develop pre-eclampsia, eclampsia, severe anemia, phlebitis, significant infection, signs of fetal intrauterine growth retardation, or other significant medical problems should discontinue participation in the exercise program.
†Adapted from Reference 15.

TABLE 11–7. CONTRAINDICATIONS FOR EXERCISING DURING PREGNANCY*

1. Pregnancy induced hypertension
2. Pre-term rupture of membrane
3. Pre-term labor during the prior or current pregnancy
4. Incompetent cervix
5. Persistent second to third trimester bleeding
6. Intrauterine growth retardation

*Reprinted with permission from Reference 14.

criterion measure of intensity, since the 15 to 20 beat/min increase in resting maternal HR make the standard training HR formulas ineffective. Also, in the previously published guidelines, maternal core temperature was not to exceed 38° C. However, recent human studies have found no evidence of fetal distress or abnormalities associated with normally increased core temperatures observed during exercise.

ACOG guidelines now differentiate between women who exercise and become pregnant and women who start exercising during pregnancy. ACOG recommends that women who currently participate in a regular exercise program can continue their training during pregnancy. Studies have demonstrated that women naturally decrease their exercise duration and intensity as their pregnancy advances. Those who begin an exercise program after becoming pregnant are advised to receive physician authorization and begin exercising with low-intensity, low- (or non-) impact activities, such as walking and swimming.

THE BENEFITS OF EXERCISE DURING PREGNANCY

There is no objective evidence that a woman who exercises has shorter or less complicated labor and delivery. However, studies have shown that women who exercise regularly return to their pre-pregnancy weight, strength, and flexibility levels faster than their sedentary counterparts. And while strenuous exercise may be associated with delivery of lighter birth weight babies, these deliveries are well within normal limits. In general, sensible amounts of exercise are beneficial, but excessive exercise could compromise fetal well-being. The following are commonly cited as benefits of exercising during pregnancy:

- Reduces the severity and frequency of back pain associated with pregnancy by helping maintain better body posture
- Provides a psychological "lift" that helps counteract the feelings of stress, anxiety, and/or depression that frequently occur during pregnancy
- Helps control weight gain
- Improves digestion and reduces constipation
- Produces a greater energy reserve for meeting the requirements of daily life
- Reduces "postpartum belly"

REFERENCES

1. Ross JG and Gilbert GG: The national children and youth fitness study: A summary of findings. *JOPERD 56*:45–50, 1985.
2. Ross JG and Pate RR: The national children and youth fitness study II: A summary of findings. *JOPERD 58*:51–56, 1987.
3. American College of Sports Medicine: Opinion statement on physical fitness in children and youth. *Med Sci Sports Exerc 20*:422–423, 1988.
4. AAHPERD: *The AAHPERD Physical Best Program*. Reston, VA: American Alliance for Health, Physical Education, Recreation and Dance, 1988.
5. Chrysler Fund-Amateur Athletic Union: *Physical Fitness Program*. Bloomington, IN: The Chrysler Fund-Amateur Athletic Union, 1987.

6. *Fitnessgram User's Manual.* Dallas, TX: Institute for Aerobics Research, 1987.
7. President's Council on Physical Fitness and Sports: *The Presidential Physical Fitness Award Program.* Washington, DC: 1987.
8. American Health and Fitness Foundation: *Fit Youth Today.* Austin: American Health and Fitness Foundations, 1986.
9. American Heart Association Council on Cardiovascular Disease in the Young: *Standards for Exercise Testing in the Pediatric Age Group 66*:1377A–1397A, 1982.
10. Freedson PS, Ward A, and Rippe JM: Resistance training for youth. In *Advances in Sports Medicine and Fitness, Vol. 3.* Edited by WA Grana, JA Lombardo, BJ Sharkey, JA Stone. Chicago, IL: Yearbook Medical Publishers, 1990.
11. ACSM Resource Manual for Guidelines for Exercise Testing and Prescription, 2nd ed. Williams & Wilkins, 1993, p. 414.
12. Skinner J: *Exercise Testing and Exercise Prescription for Special Cases, 2nd Ed.* Philadelphia: Lea & Febiger, 1993.
13. Fiatarone MA, O'Neill EF, Ryan ND, et al: Exercise training and nutritional supplementation for physical frailty in very elderly people. *N Eng J Med 330*:1769–1775, 1994.
14. American College of Obstetricians and Gynecologists: *Exercise During Pregnancy and the Postpartum Period (Technical Bulletin #189).* Washington, DC: ACOG, 1994.
15. Wolfe LA, et al: Prescription of aerobic exercise during pregnancy. *Sports Med.* 8: 273–301, 1989.

appendix A

COMMON MEDICATIONS

TABLE A–1. GENERIC AND BRAND NAMES OF COMMON
DRUGS BY CLASS

Generic Name	Brand Name
Beta Blockers	
Acebutolol	Sectral
Atenolol	Tenormin
Metoprolol	Lopressor, Toprol
Nadolol	Corgard
Pindolol	Visken
Propranolol	Inderal
Timolol	Blocadren
Carteolol	Cartrol
Betaxolal	Kerlone
Bisoprolol	Zebeta
Penbutolol	Levatol
Alpha₁ Blockers	
Prazosin	Minipress
Terazosin	Hytrin
Doxazosin	Cardura

Continued on Next Page

TABLE A–1. GENERIC AND BRAND NAMES OF COMMON
DRUGS BY CLASS *Continued*

Generic Name	Brand Name
Alpha and Beta Blocker	
Labetalol	Trandate, Normodyne
Antiadrenergic Agents	
Without Selective Receptor	
Blockade	
Clonidine	Catapres
Guanabenz	Wyntensin
Guanethidine	Ismelin
Guanfacine	Tenex
Methyldopa	Aldomet
Reserpine	Serapasil
Guanadrel	Hylorel
Nitrates and Nitoglycerin	
Isosorbide dinitrate	Isordil, Diltrate
Nitroglycerin	Nitrostat, Nitrolingual spray
Nitroglycerin ointment	Nitrol ointment
Nitroglycerin patches	Transderm Nitro, Nitro-Dur II, Nitrodisc
Isosorbide mononitrate	Ismo, Monoket
Pentaerythritol tetranitrate	Cardilate
Calcium Channel Blockers	
Diltiazem	Cardizem
Nifedipine	Procardia, Adalat
Verapamil	Calan, Isoptin
Nicardipine	Cardene
Amlodipine	Norvasc
Felodipine	Plendil
Isradipine	DynaCirc
Nimodipine	Nimotop
Bepridil	Vascor
Digitalis	
Digoxin	Lanoxin

Continued on Next Page

TABLE A–1. *Continued*

Generic Name	Brand Name
Diuretics	
Thiazides	
Hydrochlorothiazide (HCTZ)	Esidrix
"Loop"	
Furosemide	Lasix
Bumetanide	Bumex
Ethacrynic acid	Edecrin
Potassium-Sparing	
Spironolactone	Aldactone
Triamterene	Dyrenium
Amiloride	Midamor
Combinations	
Triamterene and hydrochlorothiazide	Dyazide, Maxzide
Amiloride and hydrochlorothiazide	Moduretic
Others	
Metolazone	Zaroxolyn
Peripheral Vasodilators (Nonadrenergic)	
Hydralazine	Apresoline
Minoxidil	Loniten
Angiotensin-Converting Enzyme (ACE) Inhibitors	
Captopril	Capoten
Enalapril	Vasotec
Lisinopril	Prinivil, Zestril
Ramipril	Altace
Benazepril	Lotensin
Fosinopril	Monopril
Quinapril	Accupril

Continued on Next Page

TABLE A–1.   GENERIC AND BRAND NAMES OF COMMON
DRUGS BY CLASS *Continued*

Generic Name	Brand Name
Antiarrhythmic Agents	
Class I	
IA	
Quinidine	Quinidex, Quinaglute
Procainamide	Pronestyl, Procan SR
Disopyramide	Norpace
IB	
Tocainide	Tonocard
Mexiletine	Mexitil
Lidocaine	Xylocaine, Xylocard
IC	
Encainide	Enkaid
Flecainide	Tambocor
Multiclass	
Ethmozine	Moricizine
Class II	
β-Blockers	
Class III	
Amiodarone	Cordarone
Bretylium	Bretylol
Sotalol	Betapace
Class IV	
Calcium channel blockers	
Sympathomimetic Agents	
Ephedrine	Adrenalin
Epinephrine	Alupent
Metaproterenol	Proventil, Ventolin
Albuterol	Bronkosol
Isoetharine	Brethine
Cromolyn sodium	Intal

Continued on Next Page

TABLE A–1. *Continued*

Generic Name	Brand Name
Antihyperlipidemic Agents	
Cholestyramine	Questran
Colestipol	Colestid
Gemfibrozil	Lopid
Lovastatin	Mevacor
Nicotinic acid (niacin)	Nicobid, Nicolar, Slo-Niacin
Probucol	Lorelco
Pravastatin	Pravachol
Simvastatin	Zocor
Fluvastatin	Lescol
Other	
Dipyridamole	Persantine
Warfarin	Coumadin
Pentoxifylline	Trental

TABLE A–2. EFFECTS OF MEDICATIONS ON HEART RATE, BLOOD PRESSURE, THE ELECTROCARDIOGRAM (ECG), AND EXERCISE CAPACITY

Medications	Heart Rate	Blood Pressure	ECG	Exercise Capacity
I. Beta blockers (including labetalol)	↓*(R and E)	↓(R and E)	↓ HR*(R) ↓ ischemia† (E)	↑ in patients with angina; ↓ or ↔ in patients without angina
II. Nitrates	↑(R) ↑ or ↔ (E)	↓ (R) ↓ or ↔ (E)	↑ HR(R) ↑ or ↔ HR (E) ↓ ischemia†(E)	↑ in patients with angina; ↔ in patients without angina; ↑ or ↔ in patients with congestive heart failure (CHF)
III. Calcium channel blockers				
Felodipine Isradipine Nicardipine Nifedipine	↑ or ↔ (R and E)	↓ (R and E)	↑ or ↔ HR(R and E) ↓ ischemia†(E)	↑ in patients with angina; ↔ in patients without angina
Bepridil Diltiazem Verapamil	↓ (R and E)		↓ HR (R and E) ↓ ischemia† (E)	

Continued on Next Page

246

TABLE A-2. Continued

Medications	Heart Rate	Blood Pressure	ECG	Exercise Capacity
IV. Digitalis	↓ in patients w/atrial fibrillation and possibly CHF. No significantly altered in patients w/sinus rhythm	↔	May produce nonspecific ST-T wave changes (R). May produce ST segment depression (E)	Improved only in patients with atrial fibrillation or in patients with (CHF)
V. Diuretics	↔	↔ or ↓ (R and E)	↔ (R). May cause PVCs and "false positive" test results if hypokalemia occurs. May cause PVCs if hypomagnesemia occurs (E)	↔, except possibly in patients with CHF
VI. Vasodilators, nonadrenergic	↑ or ↔ (R and E)	↓ (R and E)	↑ or ↔ HR (R and E)	↔, except ↑ or ↔ in patients with CHF
ACE inhibitors	↔	↓ (R and E)	↔	↔, except ↑ or ↔ in patients with CHF
Alpha-adrenergic blockers	↔	↓ (R and E)	↔	↔

Continued on Next Page

247

TABLE A–2. *Continued*

Medications	Heart Rate	Blood Pressure	ECG	Exercise Capacity
Anti-adrenergic agents without selective blockade of peripheral receptors	↓ or ↔ (R and E)	↓ (R and E)	↓ or ↔ HR (R and E)	↔
VII. Antiarrhythmic agents		All antiarrhythmic agents may cause new or worsened arrhythmias (proarrhythmic effect)		
Class I Quinidine Disopyramide	↑ or ↔ (R and E)	↓ or ↔ (R) ↔ (E)	↑ or ↔ HR (R) May prolong QRS and QT intervals (R) Quinidine may result in "false negative" test results (E)	↔
Procainamide	↔	↔	May prolong QRS and QT intervals (R) May result in "false positive" test results (E)	↔

Continued on Next Page

	Heart Rate	Blood Pressure	ECG	Exercise Capacity
Phenytoin Tocainide Mexiletine	↔	↔	↔	↔
Flecainide Moricizine	↔	↔	May prolong QRS and QT intervals (R) ↔ (E)	↔
Class II Beta blockers (see I.)				
Propafenone	↓ HR (R) ↓ or ↔ HR (E)	↓ (R) ↓ or ↔ (E)	↔	↔
Class III Amiodarone	↓ HR (R) ↔ (E)	↓ (R and E)	↔	↔
Class IV Calcium channel blockers (see III.)				
VIII. Bronchodila- tors	↔	↔	↔	Bronchodilators ↑ exercise capacity in patients limited by bronchospasm
Anticholinergic agents Methylxanthines	↑ or ↔ HR May produce PVCs (R and E)	↑ or ↔ (R and E)	↔	↔

Continued on Next Page

TABLE A–2. *Continued*

Medications	Heart Rate	Blood Pressure	ECG	Exercise Capacity
Sympathomimetic agents	↑ or ↔ (R and E)	↑, ↔, or ↓ (R and E)	↑ or ↔ HR (R and E)	↔
Cromolyn sodium	↔	↔	↔	↔
Corticosteroids	↔	↔	↔	↔
IX. Hyperlipidemic agents	Clofibrate may provoke arrhythmias, angina in patients with prior myocardial infarction Dextrothyroxine may ↑ HR and BP at rest and during exercise, provoke arrhythmias, and worsen myocardial ischemia and angina Nicotinic acid may ↓ BP Probucol may cause QT interval prolongation All other hyperlipidemic agents have no effect on HR, BP, and ECG			↔
X. Psychotropic medications Minor tranquilizers	May ↓ HR and BP by controlling anxiety. No other effects.			
Antidepressants	↑ or ↔ (R and E)	↓ or ↔	Variable (R) May result in "false positive" test results (E)	
Major tranquilizers	↑ or ↔ (R and E)	↓ or ↔	Variable (R) May result in "false positive" or "false negative" test results (E)	

Continued on Next Page

TABLE A-2. Continued

Lithium	↔	↔	May result in T wave changes and arrhythmias (R and E)	
XI. Nicotine	↑ or ↔ (R and E)	↑ (R and E)	↑ or ↔ HR, May provoke ischemia, arrhythmias (R and E)	↔, except ↓ or ↔ in patients with angina
XII. Antihistamines	↔	↔	↔	↔
XIII. Cold medications with sympathomimetic agents	Effects similar to those described in sympathomimetic agents, although magnitude of effects is usually smaller			
XIV. Thyroid medications Only levothyroxine	↑ (R and E)	↑ (R and E)	↑ HR May provoke arrhythmias ↑ ischemia (R and E)	↔, unless angina worsened
XV. Alcohol	↔	Chronic use may have role in ↑ BP (R and E)	May provoke arrhythmias (R and E)	↔
XVI. Hypoglycemic agents Insulin and oral agents	↔	↔	↔	↔

Continued on Next Page

TABLE A–2. Continued

Medications	Heart Rate	Blood Pressure	ECG	Exercise Capacity
XVII. Dipyridamole	↔	↔	↔	↔
XVIII. Anticoagulants	↔	↔	↔	↔
XIX. Anti-gout medications	↔	↔	↔	↔
XX. Antiplatelet medications	↔	↔	↔	↔
XXI. Pentoxifylline	↔	↔	↔	↑ or ↔ in patients limited by intermittent claudication
XXII. Caffeine	Variable effects depending upon previous use Variable effects on exercise capacity May provoke arrhythmias			
XXIII. Diet pills	↑ or ↔	↑ or ↔	↑ or ↔ HR	

Key:↑ = increase, ↔ = no effect, ↓ = decrease.
*Beta-blockers with ISA lower resting HR only slightly.
†May prevent or delay myocardial ischemia (see text).
R = rest; E = exercise.

appendix B

EMERGENCY MANAGEMENT

The following key points are essential components of all emergency medical plans:

- All personnel involved with exercise testing and supervision should be trained in basic cardiopulmonary resuscitation (CPR) and preferably Advanced Cardiac Life Support (ACLS)
- Telephone numbers for emergency assistance should be clearly posted on all telephones. Emergency communication devices must be readily available and working properly
- Emergency plans should be established and posted. Regular rehearsal of emergency plans and scenarios should be conducted and documented
- Regular drills should be conducted at least quarterly for all personnel

If a problem occurs during exercise testing, the nearest physician available should be immediately summoned. The physician should make the decision whether or not to call for evacuation to the nearest hospital if testing is not carried out in the hospital. If a physician is not available and there is any question as to the status of the patient, then emergency transportation to the closest hospital should immediately be summoned.

TABLE B–1. EMERGENCY EQUIPMENT AND DRUGS

Equipment

Defibrillator-monitor
Airway equipment
Oxygen
AMBU bag with pressure release valve
Suction equipment
Intravenous sets and stand
Intravenous fluids
Syringes and needles in multiple sizes
Adhesive tape

Drugs (IV form unless otherwise indicated)

Lidocaine
Epinephrine
Atropine
Isoproterenol
Procainamide
Sodium bicarbonate
Bretylium
Verapamil
Propranolol or Esmolol
Diazepam
Dopamine
Digoxin
Adenosine
Dobutamine
Nitroglycerine
Furosemide
Nitroglycerine tablets and/or oral spray

Equipment and drugs that should be available in any area where maximal exercise testing is performed are listed in Table B–1. Only those personnel authorized by law to use certain equipment (e.g., defibrillators, syringes, needles) and dispense drugs can lawfully do so.

Tables B–2 through B–4 provide sample plans for non-emergency situations (Table B–2) and emergency situations (B–3 and B–4). These plans are provided only as examples and specific plans must be tailored to individual program needs.

TABLE B–2. PLAN FOR NONEMERGENCY SITUATIONS

Level: Basic	Intermediate	High
At a field, pool, or park without emergency equipment	At a gymnasium or outside facility with basic equipment plus defibrillator and possibly a small "start-up" kit with drugs	Hospital or hospital-adjunct with all the equipment of intermediate level plus a "code cart" containing emergency drugs and equipment for intravenous drug administration, intubation, drawing arterial blood gas samples, and suctioning.
	Victim may be inpatient or outpatient	

Continued on Next Page

TABLE B–2. PLAN FOR NONEMERGENCY SITUATIONS *Continued*

Level: Basic	Intermediate	High
First Rescuer	**First Rescuer**	**First Rescuer**

1. Instruct victim to stop activity
2. Remain with victim until symptoms subside
  a. If symptoms worsen, use basic first aid
  b. If symptoms do not subside, bring victim to ER or MD office for evaluation
3. Advise victim to seek medical advice before further activity
	Same as Basic level No. 1–3
	Add:
	4. Take vital signs
	5. Monitor and record rhythm
	6. Bring record of vital signs and strip to ER/MD office if symptoms do not subside and visit is necessary
		Inpatient facility
		Same as Intermediate level No. 1–5
		Add:
		6. Call for RN if on ward for RN or MD if in clinic to evaluate
		7. Notify primary MD
		8. Documentation
		9. Request new consult from MD to resume exercise if more than 3 consecutive exercise sessions are interrupted for same complaint

Second Rescuer	**Second Rescuer**	**Second Rescuer**
1. Assist First Rescuer, drive victim to ER or MD office if necessary	Same as Basic level No. 1 Add: 2. Bring BP cuff, monitor to site 3. Assist with taking and monitoring vital signs	Same as Intermediate level No. 1–3

TABLE B–3. PLAN FOR POTENTIALLY LIFE-THREATENING
SITUATIONS

Level: Basic	Intermediate	High
At a field, pool, or park without emergency equipment	At a gymnasium or outside facility with basic equipment plus defibrillator and possibly a small "start-up" kit with drugs	Hospital or hospital-adjunct with all the equipment of intermediate level plus a "code cart" containing emergency drugs and equipment for intravenous drug administration, intubation, drawing arterial blood gas samples, and suctioning
	Victim may be inpatient or outpatient	

Level: Basic	Intermediate	High
First Rescuer	**First Rescuer**	**First Rescuer**

1. Establish responsiveness
  a. Responsive:
   Instruct victim to sit
   Call for help
   Direct Second Rescuer to call EMS
   Stay with victim until EMS team arrives
   Note time of incident
   Apply pressure to any bleeding
   Note if victim takes any medication (i.e., nitroglycerin)
   Take pulse
	Same as Basic level No. 1 and No. 2
	Add:
	3. Apply monitor to victim and record rhythm. Monitor continuously
	4. Take vital signs every 1 to 5 minutes
	5. Document vital signs and rhythm. Note time, and victim signs and symptoms
		Same as Intermediate level No. 1–5
		
		Also may adapt/add:
		1. Call RN on ward
		2. Call RN if MD is off ward
		3. Notify primary MD as soon as possible

Continued on Next Page

TABLE B–3. PLAN FOR POTENTIALLY LIFE-THREATENING SITUATIONS *Continued*

Level: Basic	Intermediate	High
First Rescuer	**First Rescuer**	**First Rescuer**

b. Unresponsive:
   Place victim supine
   Open airway
   Call for help
   Check respiration. If absent, follow directions in Table B–4
   Maintain open airway
   Check pulse. If absent follow directions in Table B–4
   Direct Second Rescuer to call EMS
   Stay with victim; continue to monitor respiration and pulse
2. Other considerations
  a. If bleeding, compress area to decrease/stop bleeding
  b. Suspected neck fracture: open airway with a jaw-thrust maneuver. Do not hyperextend neck		

Continued on Next Page

TABLE B–3. *Continued*

Level: Basic	Intermediate	High
First Rescuer	**First Rescuer**	**First Rescuer**
c. If seizing: prevent injury by removing harmful objects. Place something under head if possible. Turn victim on side once seizure activity stops to help drain secretions		
Second Rescuer	**Second Rescuer**	**Second Rescuer**
1. Call EMS 2. Wait to direct emergency team to scene, then 3. Return to scene to assist	Same as Basic level No. 1–3 4. Bring all emergency equipment and a. Place victim on monitor b. Run strips c. Take vital signs	Same as Intermediate level No. 1–4
Third Rescuer	**Third Rescuer**	**Third Rescuer**
1. Direct emergency team to scene or 2. Assist First Rescuer	Same as Basic level No. 1 and 2	Same as Basic level No. 1 and 2

TABLE B–4. PLAN FOR LIFE-THREATENING SITUATIONS

Level: Basic	Intermediate	High
At a field, pool, or park without emergency equipment	At a gymnasium or outside facility with basic equipment plus defibrillator and possibly a small "start-up" kit with drugs	Hospital or hospital-adjunct with all the equipment of intermediate level plus a "code cart" containing emergency drugs and equipment for intravenous drug administration, intubation, drawing arterial blood gas samples, and suctioning.
	Victim may be inpatient or outpatient	

Level: Basic	Intermediate	High
First Rescuer	**First Rescuer**	**First Rescuer**
1. Position victim (pull from pool if necessary) and place supine, determine unresponsiveness 2. Call for help (911 or local EMS number) 3. Open airway; look, listen, and feel for the air 4. Give 2 ventilations if no respirations 5. Check pulse (carotid artery) 6. Administer 15:2 compression/ventilation if no pulse 7. Continue ventilation if no respiration	Step No. 1–7 for Basic level	Step No. 1–7 of Basic level

Continued on Next Page

Second Rescuer	Second Rescuer	Second Rescuer

1. Locate nearest phone and call EMS
2. Return to scene and help with 2-person CPR, or
3. Remain at designated area and direct emergency team to location
	Step No. 1–3 of Basic Level
	Add:
	4. Return to scene, bringing defibrillator: take "quick look" at rhythm. Document rhythm [do not defibrillate unless certified to do so and this activity is part of your clinical privileges for the facility in which the work is being completed]
	5. Place monitor leads on patient and monitor rhythm during CPR
	6. Bring emergency drug kit if available
	   a. Open oxygen equipment and use AMBU bag with oxygen at 10L [if trained to do so]
	   b. Open drug kit and prepare intravenous line and drug administration [must only be done by trained, licensed professionals]
	   c. Keep equipment at scene for use by emergency personnel
		Step No. 1–6 of Intermediate level

Continued on Next Page

TABLE B–4. PLAN FOR LIFE-THREATENING SITUATIONS
Continued

Third Rescuer	Third Rescuer	Third Rescuer
1. Assist with 2-person CPR or 2. Help direct emergency team to site 3. Help clear area	Same as Basic Level	Step No. 1–3 of Basic level

appendix C

ECG INTERPRETATION AND RELATED DIAGNOSTIC INFORMATION

The tables in this Appendix are designed to provide a quick reference source for ECG recording and interpretation and for serum concentrations of enzymes commonly used as indices of myocardial necrosis. Each of these tables should be used as part of the overall clinical picture when making diagnostic decisions about an individual client or patient.

TABLE C–1. PRECORDIAL (CHEST) LEAD ELECTRODE PLACEMENT

Lead	Electrode Placement
V_1	On the right sternal border in the 4th intercostal space
V_2	On the left sternal border in the 4th intercostal space
V_3	At the midpoint of a straight line between V_2 and V_4
V_4	On the midclavicular line in the 5th intercostal space
V_5	On the anterior axillary line and horizontal to V_4
V_6	On the midaxillary line and horizontal to V_4 and V_5

TABLE C–2. ECG INTERPRETATION STEPS

1. Calculate heart rate
2. Determine the rhythm
3. Calculate intervals (PR, QRS, QT)
4. Determine the mean QRS axis and T wave axis
5. Examine ST segments and look for abnormal ($\geq$0.04 sec) Q waves
6. Look for a QRS wave transition zone between V_1 and V_6 and any obvious signs of hypertrophy
7. Develop an interpretation consistent with any abnormal values in steps 1 through 6

TABLE C–3. THE RESTING 12-LEAD ECG: NORMAL LIMITS

Parameter	Normal Limits	If abnormal, ...	Possible Interpretation(s)*
Heart rate	60 to 100 bpm	<60	Bradycardia
		>100	Tachycardia
PR interval	0.12<PR <0.20 sec	≤0.12	Accelerated conduction, e.g., W-P-W, L-G-L
			Nonsinus (low atrial) beat
		≥0.20	1° AV block
QRS interval	<0.12 sec	Look at V_1, V_6	RBBB, LBBB
			Drug/electrolyte changes
			Aberrant conduction
		Look for delta wave; is there a P wave?	W-P-W
			PVC
QT interval	>0.44 (but rate dependent; see Table C–4)	Check clinical status	Drug/electrolyte changes
QRS axis	–30°<QRS<110°	≤–30°	LAD
		≥110°	RAD
T axis	Generally same direction as QRS axis		Ischemia, subendocardial MI
ST segments	Frontal plane, $V_{5–6}$: ±1 mm V_1–V_4: <3 mm elevation <1 mm depression		Myocardial injury
Q waves	<0.04 sec		Transmural MI
Transition zone	Present between V_1 and V_6		RVH Anterior MI

*If supported by other ECG and related diagnostic criteria.

TABLE C–4. NORMAL VALUES FOR THE QT INTERVAL AS A
FUNCTION OF HEART RATE

Heart Rate (beats/min)	QT Interval (sec)
40	0.42–0.50
50	0.36–0.46
60	0.33–0.43
70	0.30–0.40
80	0.29–0.38
90	0.28–0.36
100	0.27–0.35
110	0.27–0.35
120	0.25–0.32
150	0.23–0.28

TABLE C–5. LOCALIZING AND NAMING TRANSMURAL
INFARCTS

Significant Q Waves in	Infarct Location
V_1–V_2	Anteroseptal
V_2–V_4	Anterior
V_5–V_6	Anterolateral
V_1–V_6	Extensive anterior
V_5–V_6, I, aVL	High lateral
II, III, aVF	Inferior
R>S in V_1	Posterior

TABLE C-6. SUPRAVENTRICULAR VS. VENTRICULAR ECTOPIC BEATS

Parameter	Supraventricular (Normal conduction)	Supraventricular (Aberrant conduction)	Ventricular
QRS Complex Duration	<0.12 sec	≥0.12 sec (but typically <0.15 sec)	≥0.12 sec
Configuration	Normal	Abnormal; usually has same initial vector as normal beats and pattern is often triphasic	Abnormal; pattern may be biphasic or triphasic
P wave	May be present or absent	May be present or absent	Absent
Rhythm	No compensatory pause	No compensatory pause	Often followed by compensatory pause

267

TABLE C–7. SERUM ENZYMES (MYOCARDIAL TISSUE NECROSIS)

Enzyme	Normal Value	Time Course of Change (when abnormally elevated)
Aspartate aminotransferase (AST; also called SGOT)	(<45 U/ml)	Appears within hours and peaks between 12 to 24 h; returns to normal over next several days
Creatinine phosphokinase (CPK or CK)	(<30 U/ml)	Appears within hours and peaks within 24 h; returns to normal within 3 to 5 days
CK Myocardial Band (CK–MB) or	(<5% CK)	Appears at 4 to 6 hours; peaks 12 to 24 h; returns to normal within 48 h
Lactate dehydrogenase (LDH)	(<600 U/ml)	Rises within 12 to 24 h, and peaks by day 3; returns to normal in 8 to 12 days

METABOLIC CALCULATIONS

DIRECT CALORIMETRY

A fundamental aspect of exercise testing and prescription is the ability to measure or estimate energy expenditure during exercise. Since exercise, like all metabolic events, produces heat, the rate of heat produced is directly proportional to the energy expended. However, *direct calorimetry*—the measurement of heat production is difficult to accomplish in exercising humans for a number of reasons:

- The necessary equipment, a large airtight chamber with very rigid engineering requirements, is expensive and not readily available
- When humans exercise, not all heat produced is liberated. Some is stored in the body as core temperature rises

- Many exercise ergometers (e.g., a motor driven treadmill) give off heat from their own energy transformations
- Sweating, and evaporation of sweat into the environment, affects the constants involved in the heat balance equations, which in turn affects accuracy of measurement

INDIRECT CALORIMETRY

For those reasons, the rate of energy expenditure during exercise is typically measured by *indirect calorimetry*—by measuring the rate of oxygen uptake ($\dot{V}O_2$) of the exercising individual. In this notation, the V stands for volume, the O_2 for oxygen, and the dot above the V denotes a rate, that is, a volume of oxygen per unit of time. In order for $\dot{V}O_2$ to accurately reflect energy expenditure, the exercise must be primarily aerobic. Any large proportion of anaerobic metabolism will result in an error in the measurement of energy expenditure. For this reason, $\dot{V}O_2$ measurement is usually reserved for steady state activities lasting a minimum of 90 seconds.

$\dot{V}O_2$ provides much useful information for exercise professionals:

- Under certain conditions, $\dot{V}O_2$ provides a measure of the energy cost of exercise
- The rate of oxygen uptake during maximal exercise ($\dot{V}O_{2max}$) indicates the capacity for oxygen transport and utilization during exercise
- $\dot{V}O_{2max}$ also serves as the criterion measure of aerobic fitness for inter- and intra-individual comparisons
- In combination with the measured rate of carbon dioxide output ($\dot{V}CO_2$), $\dot{V}O_2$ provides general information about the fuels being used for exercise

Various standard units are used for $\dot{V}O_2$ depending on the purpose for its measurement:

- The absolute rate of oxygen uptake is typically given by the units liters per minute **(L/min)**. In this form, $\dot{V}O_2$ can be directly converted to a rate of energy expenditure. These units (or more typically ml/min) are also used in estimating the energy cost of non-weightbearing activities, such as cycle or arm ergometry
- For comparing the $\dot{V}O_2$ of individuals who vary in body size and for estimating the energy cost of weightbearing aerobic activities (such as treadmill walking, running, or bench stepping), milliliters per kg of body weight per minute **(ml · kg^{-1} · min^{-1})** are the preferred units
- A third important set of units for $\dot{V}O_2$ is **ml · kg FFW^{-1} · min^{-1}**. Here, FFW refers to the fat-free weight of the individual. When the purpose of measuring $\dot{V}O_2$ is to assess cardiopulmonary function, these units may be preferable to ml · kg^{-1} · min^{-1}, since the latter are sensitive to changes in body weight, and especially fatness, independent of any alteration in the capacity of the cardiopulmonary system

MEASUREMENT OF $\dot{V}O_2$

The actual measurement of $\dot{V}O_2$ is typically performed in laboratory or clinical settings using a procedure called *open-circuit spirometry*. Open-circuit spirometry involves the subject inspiring room air and expiring into a gas collection and measurement system. Aside from a breathing valve with mouthpiece (which provides unidirectional flow), a noseclip (which ensures that all gas exchange takes place at the mouth), and tubing involved in such a system, there are three basic pieces of equipment that are necessary:

- A device that measures the volume of expired air ($\dot{V}_E$) or inspired air ($\dot{V}_I$) over a fixed period of time, such as a dry-gas meter. This volume must then be corrected to standard temperature and pressure, dry (STPD) conditions, that is, the volume which would be present if the prevailing ambient conditions were 0°C, 760 mm Hg barometric pressure, with no water vapor pressure
- An oxygen analyzer, which measures the fraction of O_2 in the expired air (F_EO_2)
- A CO_2 analyzer, which measures the fraction of CO_2 in the expired air (F_ECO_2)

These individual pieces of equipment, or similar devices, are often integrated and interfaced with a computer in commercially available metabolic units. The fractions of O_2 and CO_2 in the inspired air are constant and known [$F_IO_2 = 0.2093$ (20.93%) and $F_ICO_2 = 0.0003$ (0.03%]. $\dot{V}O_2$ (in the same units as $\dot{V}_E$) can then be calculated according to the following equation:

$$\dot{V}O_2 = \dot{V}_E \times [0.265 \times (1.000 - F_EO_2 - F_ECO_2) - F_EO_2]$$
$$= \dot{V}_I \times [0.2093 - (0.7904 \times F_EO_2) / (1.000 - F_EO_2 - F_ECO_2)]$$

RESPIRATORY EXCHANGE RATIO (R) AND RESPIRATORY QUOTIENT (RQ)

Both R and RQ are calculated as $\dot{V}CO_2/\dot{V}O_2$ and are unitless variables. While these two calculated variables are often used synonymously, there is one important distinction between the two. Since R is a ventilatory measurement, it can be measured over a very short period of time (e.g., one minute). Conversely, RQ measures cellular respiration, and implies that the measurement has been made over a longer period, typically 15 minutes or more. RQ provides information about substrate utilization at the cellular level, equaling 1.0 for pure carbohydrate oxidation, 0.7 for mixed fat oxidation, and approximately 0.8 for mixed proteins. RQ therefore always falls between 0.7 and 1.0. R, on the other hand, since it is influenced by respiratory events, can exceed 1.0 during heavy nonsteady state or maximal exercise, due to (1) hyperventilation (which disproportionately increases $\dot{V}CO_2$), and (2) buffering of lactic acid in the blood.

ESTIMATION OF ENERGY EXPENDITURE—METABOLIC CALCULATIONS

When it is not possible or feasible to measure $\dot{V}O_2$, reasonably accurate estimates can still be made for steady state exercise. Regression equations have been derived from laboratory data relating mechanical measures of work rate and their metabolic equivalents. These equations are appropriate for general clinical and laboratory usage when standard ergometric devices are available but spirometry is not. They also have utility for estimating or predicting energy expenditure (and thus weight loss) for some nonergometer exercise modalities (e.g., indoor or outdoor walking or running). Several cautionary notes about the use of metabolic calculations are in order:

- The measured $\dot{V}O_2$ at a given work rate is highly reproducible for a given individual; however, the intersubject variability in measured $\dot{V}O_2$ may have a standard error of estimate (SEE) as high as 7%. Since the equations are often used to predict $\dot{V}O_2$, it is important to remember that the variance of a predicted value is much larger than the SEE (i.e., the prediction interval is greater than the confidence interval)
- As noted above, these equations are appropriate only for steady state submaximal aerobic exercise. Failure to achieve a steady state will result in an overestimation of $\dot{V}O_2$
- While the accuracy of these equations is unaffected by most environmental influences (heat and cold), anything that changes the mechanical efficiency (gait abnormalities; wind, snow, or sand) will result in a loss of accuracy
- Inherent assumptions for the use of the equations presuppose that ergometers are properly calibrated and used appropriately, e.g., no rail-holding during treadmill exercise

TABLE D–1. FORMULAS FOR ESTIMATING MAXIMAL AND TARGET HEART RATES

1. **Maximal heart rate (HR_{max})**
   $HR_{max} = 220 - age$　　　　　　　　(low estimate)
   $HR_{max} = 210 - (0.5 \times age)$　　　(high estimate)
   - For each equation, the standard deviation = ±10 to 12 beats/min
2. **Target (training) heart rate**
   $HR = [exercise\ intensity \times (HR_{max} - HR_{rest})] + HR_{rest}$　　(Karvonen formula[*])
   $HR = exercise\ intensity \times (HR_{max}) \times 1.15$　　(%HR_{max} formula[†])
   - Where exercise intensity is the percentage of maximal intensity

[*]From *Am Med Exp Biol Fenn* 35:307, 1957.
[†]Since taking a straight percentage of maximal heart rate underestimates training heart rates by approximately 15%.

Despite these caveats, proper and judicious use of metabolic calculations provides a valuable tool for the exercise professional. In addition to estimates of energy expenditure, it is often necessary or desirable to estimate heart rate responses during exercise. There are several useful equations for estimating heart rate (see Table D–1).

STEPWISE APPROACH TO USING METABOLIC CALCULATIONS

While use of metabolic calculations is relatively simple and straightforward for the experienced professional, it is often a source of confusion for the novice user. Presented in this section is a stepwise approach to using these equations. While an advanced knowledge of mathematics is not necessary, the ability to solve for an unknown variable in a simple algebraic expression is essential.

Presented below is a simple 3-step procedure which facilitates easy use of metabolic calculations. It is recommended that novice users of these equations follow these steps each time.

Step 1. Conversion to appropriate units and knowledge of oommon equivalents

1. Convert all weights from pounds (lb) to kilograms (kg)
   - lb ÷ 2.2 = kg
2. Convert speed from miles per hour (mi/h) to meters per minute (m/min)
   - mi/h × 26.8 = m/min
   - (Another useful relationship is: 60 ÷ min/mile = mi/h)
3. Common equivalents:
   - liters O_2 × 5 = kilocalories (kcal)
   - 3500 kcal = approximately 1 lb of fat gain or loss
   - Vo_2 in ml · kg^{-1} · min^{-1} ÷ 3.5 = METs
   - kgm/min ÷ 6 = watts (W)

Step 2. Transform $\dot{V}O_2$ into the most appropriate units.

1. If the activity in question is weightbearing—walking, running, bench stepping—convert to $ml \cdot kg^{-1} \cdot min^{-1}$
2. If the activity in question is not weightbearing—cycling, arm ergometry—convert to ml/min
3. If the question involves caloric expenditure or weight loss, convert to L/min

---

Each metabolic equation considers three components of energy expenditure, a resting component (R), a horizontal component (H), and a vertical component (V). The sum of these three equals the entire energy cost of the activity.

Step 3. Write the appropriate equation in the form $\dot{V}O_2 = R + H + V$

Table D–2 summarizes the important steps used in calculating $\dot{V}O_2$ for various exercise modalities. Keep in mind that in practice, $\dot{V}O_2$ is often known and one of the other terms in the equation—treadmill speed or grade, cycle ergometer resistance, etc.—is the unknown variable.

Following are specific equations that are provided for various exercise modalities. After completing the previous Steps 1–3, these equations may be used where appropriate.

Walking [appropriate for speeds of 50 to 100 m/min (1.9 to 3.7 mi/h) or higher if the individual is truly walking]

1. $R = 3.5 \, ml \cdot kg^{-1} \cdot min^{-1}$ (by definition, 1 MET)

---

2. H = 0.1 × walking speed (in m/min)
   - 0.1 is the regression constant for converting m/min to ml · kg^{-1} · min^{-1}
3. V = 1.8 × speed (in m/min) × grade (as a decimal)
   - 1.8 is the constant for converting m/min to ml · kg^{-1}· min^{-1}
   - for example, 5% grade is written as 0.05 in this format
   - for walking on a level treadmill or for overground walking that begins and ends at the same point, V = 0
4. $\dot{V}O_2$ (in ml · kg^{-1}· min^{-1}) = R + H + V

This equation is more accurate for grade walking than for level walking, for which it may underestimate $\dot{V}O_2$ by as much as 15 to 20%. Also, for children and adolescents, the equation underestimates $\dot{V}O_2$ by approximately 0.5 ml · kg^{-1} · min^{-1} for each year below the age of 18.

Running (appropriate for speeds >134 m/min or 5.0 mi/h. This equation can also be used for speeds between 3 and 5 mi/h if the individual is truly running)

1. R = 3.5 ml · kg^{-1} · min^{-1} (by definition, 1 MET)
2. H = 0.2 × walking speed (in m/min)
   - 0.2 is the regression constant for converting m/min to ml · kg^{-1} · min^{-1}
3. V = 0.9 × speed (in m/min) × grade (as a decimal)
   - 0.9 is the constant for converting m/min to ml · kg^{-1}· min^{-1}
   - for example, 5% grade is written as 0.05 in this format
   - for running on a level treadmill or for outdoor running that begins and ends at the same point, V = 0. (This equation should not be used for overground running up or down grades)
4. $\dot{V}O_2$ (in ml · kg^{-1} · min^{-1}) = R + H + V

TABLE D–2. SUMMARY OF METABOLIC CALCULATIONS

$\dot{V}_{O_2}$ Mode (units)	=	Resting Component (R)	+	Horizontal Component (H)
Walking $(ml \cdot kg^{-1} \cdot min^{-1})$	=	$3.5\ ml \cdot kg^{-1} \cdot min^{-1}$	+	$m/min \times 0.1$
Running $(ml \cdot kg^{-1} \cdot min^{-1})$	=	$3.5\ ml \cdot kg^{-1} \cdot min^{-1}$	+	$m/min \times 0.2$
Leg Ergometer (ml/min)	=	$3.5\ ml \cdot kg^{-1} \cdot min^{-1} \times kg\ BW$	+	None

Continued on Next Page

TABLE D–2. *Continued*

+	Vertical or Resistive Component (V)	Comments
+	grade (frac) × m/min × 1.8	1. For speeds of 50–100 m/min (1.9–3.7 mi/h) 2. 1 mi/h = 26.8 m/min
+	grade (frac) × m/min × 0.9	1. For speeds >134 m/min (>5.0 mi/h) 2. If truly jogging (not walking), this equation can also be used for speeds between 80 and 134 m/min (3–5 mi/h) 3. Formula applies to level running off the treadmill, but not to grade running off the treadmill
+	kgm/min × 2	1. For work rates between 300–1200 kgm/min 2. $\text{kgm/min} = \text{kg} \times \dfrac{m}{rev} \times \dfrac{rev}{min}$ 3. Multiply resting component by body weight (kg) to convert to $\text{ml} \cdot \text{min}^{-1}$ 4. Monarch™ = 6 m/rev Tunturi™ = 3 m/rev BodyGuard™ = 3 m/rev

Continued on Next Page

TABLE D–2. SUMMARY OF METABOLIC CALCULATIONS
Continued

$\dot{V}O_2$ Mode (units)	=	Resting Component (R)	+	Horizontal Component (H)
Arm Ergometer (ml/min)	=	$3.5 \text{ ml} \cdot \text{kg}^{-1} \cdot \text{min}^{-1}$ $\times$ kg BW	+	None
Stepping ($\text{ml} \cdot \text{kg}^{-1} \cdot \text{min}^{-1}$)	=	Included in horizontal and vertical components	+	steps/min $\times$ 0.35

Continued on Next Page

Prediction equations have also been published based on exercise duration using standard protocols. One such equation in common use, based on the Bruce protocol, is:

$$\dot{V}O_{2max} \text{ (in ml} \cdot \text{kg}^{-1} \cdot \text{min}^{-1}) = 14.8 - (1.379 \times \text{time in min}) + (0.451 \times \text{time}^2) - (0.012 \times \text{time}^3)^*$$

*From Foster C et al. *Am Heart J. 108*:1229–1234, 1984.

It is typically desirable to test patients without the use of handrail support. However, with some patient and

TABLE D–2. *Continued*

+	Vertical or Resistive Component (V)	Comments
+	$\dfrac{kg \cdot m}{min} \times 3$	1. For work rates between 150–750 kg · m · min⁻¹ 2. $\dfrac{kg \cdot m}{min} = kg \times \dfrac{m}{rev} \times \dfrac{rev}{min}$ 3. Multiply resting component by body weight (kg) to convert to ml/min
+	$\dfrac{m}{steps} \times \dfrac{steps}{min} \times 1.33 \times 1.8$	1. 1.33 includes both positive component of going up (1.0) + negative component of going down (0.33) 2. Stepping height in meters

elderly populations this may not be possible. A validated equation has been published for use when treadmill walking is done with handrail support using the Bruce protocol:

$$\dot{V}O_{2max} \text{ (in ml} \cdot kg^{-1} \cdot min^{-1}) = (2.282 \times \text{time in min}) + 8.545^{*}$$

*From McConnell TR and Clark BA. *J. Cardiopulm. Rehab* 7:324–331, 1987.

Equations for estimating $\dot{V}O_2$ during leg and arm ergometry and stepping follow:

Leg cycle ergometry (appropriate for power outputs between 300 and 1200 kgm/min)

1. $R = 3.5 \text{ ml} \cdot \text{kg}^{-1} \cdot \text{min}^{-1} \times$ body weight in kg
   - multiplication by body weight converts $\text{ml} \cdot \text{kg}^{-1} \cdot \text{min}^{-1}$ into ml/min
2. $H = 0$
   - there is no horizontal component for this activity
3. $V = 2.0 \times$ power output (in kgm/min)
   - 2.0 is the regression constant for converting kgm/min to ml/min
   - kgm/min = kg (or kp) of resistance × meters per pedal revolution × pedal rate (rev/min)
     - kg is the resistance or "tension" setting on the ergometer
     - meters per pedal revolution is a function of the ergometer being used
       - = 6 m/rev for Monark™ ergometers
       - = 3 m/rev for Tunturi™ and BodyGuard™ ergometers
     - pedal rate must be known
       - typically 50 or 60 rpm for untrained cyclists
       - can use 80 rpm or greater for trained cyclists
     - electronic ergometers control power output independent of pedal rate
4. $\dot{V}O_2$ (in ml/min) = R + H + V, where H is 0

Arm ergometry (appropriate for power outputs between 150 and 750 kgm/min)

1. $R = 3.5 \text{ ml} \cdot \text{kg}^{-1} \cdot \text{min}^{-1} \times$ body weight in kg
   - multiplication by body weight converts $\text{ml} \cdot \text{kg}^{-1} \cdot \text{min}^{-1}$ to ml/min
2. $H = 0$
   - there is no horizontal component for this activity

3. $V = 3.0 \times$ power output (in kgm/min)
   - 3.0 is the regression constant for converting kgm/min to ml/min
   - kgm/min = kg (or kp) of resistance $\times$ meters per crank revolution $\times$ cranking rate (rev/min)
     - kg is the resistance or "tension" setting on the ergometer
     - meters per pedal revolution is a function of the ergometer being used
     - = 2.4 m/rev for Monark™ arm ergometers
     - arm cranking rate must be known
     - typically 50 or 60 rpm
4. $\dot{V}O_2$ (in ml/min) = R + H + V, where H is 0

Stepping (appropriate for power outputs between 300 and 1200 kgm/min)

1. R is already included in the H and V components of this equation
2. $H = 0.35 \times$ (steps per minute)
   - 0.35 is the regression constant for converting steps/min to $ml \cdot kg^{-1} \cdot min^{-1}$
3. V
   - for stepping up and down = 2.4 $\times$ steps/min $\times$ m/step
   - for stepping up only = 1.0 $\times$ steps/min $\times$ m/step
   - for stepping down only = 0.6 $\times$ steps/min $\times$ m/step
   - note that step height is in meters
4. $\dot{V}O_2$ (in ml kg^{-1} min^{-1}) = R + H + V, where R is 0

FIELD TEST EQUATIONS

When large numbers of individuals are being tested, or when the use of standard ergometry is not possible, field tests are commonly used to predict $\dot{V}O_{2max}$. These tests involve endurance walks or runs over level terrain designed to either (1) cover a fixed distance (such as 1 or

TABLE D–3. COMMON FIELD TEST EQUATIONS

1. **Rockport Walking Test (one mile walk)**[*]
   - $\dot{V}O_{2max}$ (in ml · kg^{-1} · min^{-1}) = 132.853 − (0.0769 × body weight) − (0.3877 × age) + (6.315 × gender) − (3.2649 × time) − (0.1565 × HR)
   - Body weight in lb; gender = 0 for female, 1 for male; time in min; HR is taken at end of walk

2. **Cooper 12-min test**[†]
   - $\dot{V}O_{2max}$ (in ml · kg^{-1} · min^{-1}) = 3.126 × (meters covered in 12 min) − 11.3

3. **Balke 15-min test**[‡]
   - $\dot{V}O_{2max}$ (in ml · kg^{-1} · min^{-1}) = 2.67 × (meters covered in 15 min) + 9.6

[*]From Kline, GM et al.: *Med Sci Sports Exerc 19*:253–259, 1987.
[†]From Cooper, K: *J Am Med Assoc 203*:201–204, 1968.
[‡]From Balke, B: Report 63-6, Federal Aviation Agency, Aeromedical Research Division, Civil Aeromedicine Research Institute, Oklahoma City, 1963.

1.5 miles) with time as the criterion measure or (2) measure the distance covered in a fixed period of time (such as 12 or 15 minutes). Some incorporate other predictor variables, such as age, gender, or body weight. Several validated field test equations are given in Table D–3.

SAMPLE METABOLIC CALCULATIONS

A 30-year-old man has a resting heart rate of 60 beats/min, weighs 180 lbs, and has a $\dot{V}O_{2max}$ of 48 ml · kg^{-1} · min^{-1}. He wishes to begin an exercise program in which he can (1) run outdoors in good weather and (2) cycle indoors during inclement weather. He owns a Monark™ mechanically braked cycle ergometer and has a flat 4-mile long trail on which he can run. You decide to begin his exercise prescription at an exercise intensity of 70% $\dot{V}O_{2max}$.

Step 1. Convert the data provided into the appropriate units

180 lb ÷ 2.2 = 81.8 kg

Step 2. Convert $\dot{V}O_2$ into the appropriate units

His exercise intensity is 0.70×48 ml $\cdot$ kg^{-1} $\cdot$ min^{-1} = 33.6 ml $\cdot$ kg^{-1} $\cdot$ min^{-1}. These are the appropriate units for running. Since he also wishes to exercise on his cycle ergometer, the $\dot{V}O_2$ should also be calculated in ml/min. This is done be multiplying 33.6 ml $\cdot$ kg^{-1} $\cdot$ min^{-1} $\times$ 81.8 kg = 2748 ml/min. If caloric expenditure is an issue, 2748 ml/min ÷ 1000 = 2.748 L/min.

Q: What is an appropriate target heart rate according to the Karvonen formula?

A: Estimated HR$_{max}$ = 220 − age
                   = 220 − 30
                   = 190 beats/min.

Target HR = [exercise intensity $\times$ (HR$_{max}$ − HR$_{rest}$)] + HR$_{rest}$
               = [0.70 $\times$ (100 − 60)] + 60
               = 151 beats/min (in practice, a range of 146 to 156 might be given, since a 10 second pulse count is recommended during exercise)

Q: What will his energy expenditure be in METs? in kcal/min?

A: 33.6 ml $\cdot$ kg^{-1} $\cdot$ min^{-1} ÷ 3.5 = 9.6 METs
   2.748 L/min $\times$ 5 = 13.7 kcal/min

Q: To exercise at the chosen intensity, how long should it take him to complete the 4-mile trail?

A: In order to calculate the exercise time, the running speed first needs to be determined.

Step 3. $\dot{V}O_2$ *(in ml · kg^{-1} · min^{-1})* = $R + H + V$
33.6 ml · kg^{-1} · min^{-1} = 3.5 ml · kg^{-1} · min^{-1} +
$$[0.2 \times (\text{speed in m/min})] + 0$$
speed = 150.5 m/min
150.5 m / min ÷ 26.8 = 5.6 mi/h
60 min/h ÷ 5.6 mi/h = 10.7 min/mi
4 miles × 10.7 min/mi = ≈ 43 min

Q: On a rainy day, what resistance setting should he use on his cycle ergometer?

A: In order to prescribe exercise on a cycle ergometer, we must predetermine a pedaling rate in rpm. In this case, we choose 60 rpm.

Step 4. $\dot{V}O_2$ *(in ml/min)* = $R + H + V$
2748 ml/min = (3.5 ml · kg^{-1} · min^{-1} × 81.8 kg) +
$$0 + (2.0 \times \text{kgm/min})$$
= 286.3 ml/min + (2.0 × kg × m/rev × rev/min)
= 286.3 ml/min + (2.0 × kg × 6 × 60)
kg resistance = 3.4 kg (or kp)

PRACTICE METABOLIC CALCULATIONS (WITH ANSWERS)

1. A man weighing 176 lb runs at a 9-minute per mile pace outdoors. What is his estimated $\dot{V}O_2$?
2. To match this exercise intensity (from #1 above) on a Tunturi^{TM} cycle ergometer, what setting would you use at a pedaling rate of 60 rev/min?
3. If this same man exercised at this intensity 5 times per week for 30 minutes each session, how long would it take him to lose 12 lb?

4. For a desired training intensity of 75% $\dot{V}O_{2max}$, at what heart rate should a 45-year-old woman exercise? Her resting heart rate is 70 beats/min.

5. A 198-lb cardiac patient wishes to use an arm ergometer for part of his rehabilitation program. He works at a power output of 300 kgm/min for 15 minutes, then at 450 kgm/min for 15 min. What is his average $\dot{V}O_2$ (in L/min) over this session?

6. If an individual reduces his or her dietary intake by 1750 kcal per week, how much weight (in lb) would he/she lose in 6 months (26 weeks)?

7. If a 13-year-old girl steps up and down on a 30-cm step at a rate of 20 steps (complete up and down cycles) per minute, what would her estimated $\dot{V}O_2$ be (in ml $\cdot$ kg^{-1} $\cdot$ min^{-1})?

8. A 71-year-old man weighing 180 lb walks on a motor-driven treadmill at 3.5 mi/h and a 15% grade. What is his estimated MET level?

ANSWERS

1. 39.2 ml $\cdot$ kg^{-1} $\cdot$ min^{-1}; 2. 7.9 kg (or kp); 3. about 18 weeks; 4. 148 to 150 beats/min; 5. 1.44 L/min; 6. 13 lb; 7. 21.4 ml $\cdot$ kg^{-1} $\cdot$ min^{-1}; 8. 10.9 METs.

ENVIRONMENTAL CONSIDERATIONS

HEAT AND HUMIDITY

Of the many environmental factors that can impact on safe and effective exercise, none is as potentially life- and health-threatening as heat stress. No well-accepted standard exists for determining safe upper temperature and humidity limits for fitness or clinical exercise environments. However, proposed heat stress guidelines exist[1-4] which provide quantitative information that can be directly applied to exercise settings. These guidelines are aimed at preventing body temperatures from rising excessively during physical exertion, mitigating the deleterious effects of dehydration, etc., and are based upon accurate assessment of (1) exercise intensity and (2) environmental conditions (either indoor or outdoor).

When trying to make decisions about exercise environments, it is important to evaluate all aspects of the environment that impact on the participant. Not only are temperature and humidity important, but air movement and (when exercising outdoors) solar radiation from sunlight also play major roles. One single temperature index which takes all these effects into account is the *wet-bulb globe temperature or WBGT*. WBGT is a single temperature which is dependent upon air temperature, humidity, solar radiation, and wind velocity, and thus represents a composite measure of the impact of the environment on exercising subjects. WBGT can be measured using relatively simple low-cost instrumentation or can be calculated from data available from local weather services, and can be expressed in either °C or °F. Three measurements are combined into the WBGT calculation—air temperature, natural wet-bulb temperature (measured by placing a wetted wick over the thermometer bulb), and globe temperature (the temperature inside a copper globe painted flat black). WBGT is calculated as:

- (Indoor) WBGT = (0.7 × natural wet-bulb temperature) + (0.3 × globe temperature)
- (Outdoor) WBGT = (0.7 × natural wet-bulb temperature) + (0.2 × globe temperature) + (0.1 × air temperature)

It is important to remember that the suggested cut-offs which follow should be used only as helpful guidelines in deciding such issues as when it is too hot to exercise, how long exercise should last under certain conditions, etc. For exercise programs and individual exercise prescription, the criteria document proposed by NIOSH [under the Occupational Safety and Health Act of 1970 (Public Law 9–596)] in 1972 and revised in 1986[1] can be adapted. Decisions about heat stress are made using 2 criteria—a *Recommended Alert Limit (RAL,* above which specific actions should be taken to reduce the effects of heat stress) and a *Ceiling Limit (C,* above which exercise should not be attempted without somehow changing the environment). Figure E–1 graphically illustrates the NIOSH approach to heat stress evaluation. Several distinct limits are presented which are based on exercise

FIG. E–1. NIOSH Recommended Heat Stress Alert (RAL) and Ceiling (C) Limits (see text for description).*

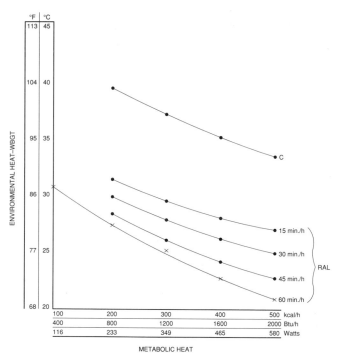

*Assumes 70 kg (154 lb) body weight and 1.8 m² (19.4 ft²) body surface.

intensity (expressed here as energy expenditure per hour) and ambient WBGT (in both °C and °F). Several RAL's are provided for intermittent exercise.

Probably the most important environmental question with which an exercise professional may be confronted is how to deal with environments below C but above the RAL. This area represents environmental conditions in which exercise can still be performed, but with increased risk to the participant. In such cases, the following actions are recommended:

- Change the environment. If the exercise area cannot be cooled to an appropriate WBGT by means of fans or air conditioning, move to an area meeting the WBGT requirements; and/or,
- For this session, decrease the exercise intensity. Like cooling the environment, lowering the intensity represents another way of staying within an acceptable temperature/intensity zone. Ways to accomplish this, while still getting a training effect include slowing the pace of exercise appropriately or making the exercise intermittent by adding rest cycles. Perhaps the most useful guide is the proper use of target heart rate (unchanged from cool conditions). Exercise heart rate is increased about 1 beat/min for every degree Centigrade above 25°C and 2 beats/min for every mm Hg above 20 mm Hg water vapor pressure. Strict adherence to a scientifically determined target rate will cause an appropriate decrease in intensity

---

One of the best means of decreasing the risk of exercise program participants developing heat illness is through a gradual acclimation to exercise in hot environments. Through this process, heart rate and body temperature at a given exercise intensity decrease, sweating rate increases, and the sweat becomes more dilute. It has been estimated that as much as 25% of the apparently healthy population may be heat intolerant in the unacclimated state, with that number decreasing to about 2% after thorough acclimation. The best method of acclimation is to aerobically exercise in a hot environment. The first such session may last as little as 10 to 15 minutes for safety reasons and gradually increase in duration to a full exercise session. It takes most healthy people 10 to 14 days to fully acclimate, although illness and alcohol consumption have been shown to slow this process. Along with heat acclimation, adequate hydration is the key to preventing untoward effects of exercise when the temperature and/or humidity are high. Progressive dehydration occurs during exercise when sweating is profuse. As little as a 2% reduction in body weight during exercise can result in impaired temperature regulation. Furthermore, a 4% decrease in body weight translates into a 6% decrease in maximal aerobic capacity and a 12% reduction in exercise time.[5]

Exercise programs should be structured around fluid availability so that participants can drink before, during, and after exercise. Participants should be encouraged to drink as much water as is physically comfortable (minimally 2 cups) 15 to 20 minutes prior to exercise, a cupful of water every 15 minutes during exercise, and more water than thirst dictates after exercise. Each pound of weight lost should be replaced with 16 oz. of fluid. This latter point is especially applicable for those participants over the age of 60, since there is a decreased thirst sensitivity to body hydration status in this age group. The fluid should be cold (45 to 55°F) and palatable, and with a few exceptions, water is the replacement drink of choice. There is little need to replace electrolytes lost during most brief exercise sessions since these small decrements are typically replenished when the next meal is eaten. For participants on a restricted salt diet, their physician should be consulted with regard to salt balance. Unless the exercise bout lasts in excess of 60 to 90 minutes, there is little advantage in supplementing carbohydrates.

The preceding guidelines assume that the exercise participant is free of any overt disease or condition which may increase the likelihood of heat illness. Many such conditions exist, including (but not limited to): hypertension (alters control of skin blood flow),[6] diabetes (neuropathies may affect sweating and/or skin blood flow), aging (alters peripheral cardiovascular and sweating responses),[7] various drug regimens (including diuretics, β-blockers, α-agonists, and vasodilators), alcohol use (causes vasodilation and enhances dehydration), obesity, and a prior history of heat illness or difficulty acclimating to heat. The exercise professional should be knowledgeable about the effects of each of these on temperature regulation.

In dealing with current or expected periods of hot weather, fitness facilities should standardize a heat stress management plan. Topics for inclusion in such a plan are:

- Increased medical screening and surveillance of participants
- Evaluation of all aspects of the thermal environment, preferably using WBGT as a criterion measure
- An approved decision-making flowchart based on proposed standards such as NIOSH, ACGIH, AIHA, etc., and tailored to your clientele and exercise setting
- Gradual acclimation policy for participants
- Provision of cold, palatable fluids and plan for increasing fluid intake before, during, and after exercise (structured drink breaks for entire group)
- Participant education, including early signs and symptoms of heat illness (chills, lightheadedness, dizziness, piloerection, nausea, etc.)
- Emergency procedures for heat illness incorporated into an overall emergency plan for the facility

COLD TEMPERATURES

In most circumstances cold presents less of an immediate health risk for exercising clients or patients. This is because most people dress appropriately (or even overdress) for outdoor exercise in cold weather and because aerobic exercise itself generates large amounts of heat. There are three primary areas of concern which the exercise professional should keep in mind:

- Prevention of frostbite and other exposure injuries
- Subjective sensation of symptoms by angina patients. Cold air breathing and dramatic skin cooling may make it more difficult for angina patients to discern and/or grade their anginal symptoms
- Cold may lower the anginal threshold or even cause angina at rest

---

Even extremely cold inspired air is adequately warmed by the airways and causes no injury to the lungs; however, there is evidence that patients breathing cold air may have difficulty noticing the onset of anginal pressure or pain.

ACUTE ALTITUDE EXPOSURE

With increasing altitude, F_IO_2 remains constant at 0.2093, but barometric pressure decreases, resulting in a reduction in P_IO_2 and possibly P_aO_2 and S_aO_2. Cardiac and pulmonary patients may travel to mountainous regions of the world where they may encounter altitudes of 3,000 to 10,000 feet or higher. Furthermore, travel in pressurized cabins of commercial airliners exposes flyers to reduced barometric pressures equivalent to an altitude of 5,000 to 8,000 feet.

The most obvious change during physical activity at high altitude is an increased pulmonary ventilation which increases the feeling of breathlessness. The response is highly variable among individuals and may not be felt for several days. This relative hyperventilation may lead to mild respiratory alkalosis and helps to attenuate the decrease in P_aO_2. At rest and during exercise at high altitude, HR may be elevated in order to increase cardiac output and help offset the reduced S_aO_2 and maintain adequate oxygen transport. The increased resting HR is transient and returns to normal after 2 to 3 days at high altitude; however, HR_{max} may remain below its sea level value. The relative hypoxia at moderate altitude may disrupt the balance between myocardial oxygen supply and demand in patients with CAD. In patients with severe LV dysfunction, systolic myocardial function may be reduced.[8]

At an altitude of 4,000 feet, a sea level resident can expect about a 5% reduction in $\dot{V}O_{2max}$, which is typically accompanied by a similar decrease in physical work capacity. For altitudes above 4,000 feet, a further progressive decline occurs. For a given absolute exercise intensity, HR is higher at moderate altitude, but target heart rate guidelines developed at lower altitudes are still valid and should be followed. Thus, as with conditions of high heat and humidity, exercise intensity or pace will be lowered accordingly.

Additional medical concerns at high altitude include acute mountain sickness (AMS) and high altitude pulmonary edema (HAPE). HAPE is a non-cardiac form of edema which, while rare, is potentially fatal. Prompt treatment with supplemental oxygen or descent to lower altitude is required. Some patient populations with pulmonary hypertension, uncompensated CHF, unstable angina, recent MI, or severe anemia may be at greater risk when traveling to higher altitudes.[8]

REFERENCES

1. National Institute for Occupational Safety and Health: Criteria for a recommended standard . . . occupational exposure to hot environments. (DHHS NIOSH Publ. No. 86–113). US Department of Health and Human Services, Washington, DC, 1986.
2. American Conference of Governmental Industrial Hygienists: Threshold limit values for chemical substances and physical agents in the workroom environment with intended changes. ACGIH, Cincinnati, 1979.
3. American Industrial Hygiene Association: Heating and cooling for man in industry, 2nd Ed. AIHA, Akron, 1975.
4. TriServices Document: Prevention, treatment, and control of heat injury. US Army TB Med 507, 1980.
5. Sawka MN, et al: Hydration and vascular fluid shifts during exercise in the heat. *J Appl Physiol 56*:91–96, 1984.
6. Kenney WL and Kamon E: Comparative physiological responses of normotensive and essentially hypertensive men to exercise in the heat. *Eur J Appl Physiol 52*:196–201, 1984.
7. Kenney WL and Havenith G: Heat stress and age: skin blood flow and body temperature. *J Therm Biol 19*:341–344, 1993.
8. Squires RW: Moderate altitude exposure and the cardiac patient. *J Cardiopulm Rehab 5*:421–426, 1985.

appendix F

AMERICAN COLLEGE OF SPORTS MEDICINE CERTIFICATIONS

This appendix details information about ACSM certification programs, as well as a complete listing of the current knowledge bases that comprise the foundations of these certification examinations. Beginning in 1995, the various ACSM certification exams will reflect the scope of knowledge, skills, and abilities detailed in this appendix. The goals of the ACSM Committee for Certification and Education through the process of certifying personnel are to (1) enhance professionalism within the fitness, clinical, and health care arenas, and (2) increase public access to appropriate exercise services.

ACSM CERTIFICATIONS AND THE PUBLIC

The first of ACSM's Clinical Track certifications was initiated nearly 20 years ago in conjunction with publication of the first edition of the *Guidelines for Exercise Testing and Prescription*. That era was marked by rapid development of exercise programs for stable coronary artery disease (CAD) patients. ACSM sought a means to disseminate accurate information on this health care initiative through expression of consensus from its members in basic science, clinical practice, and education. Thus, these early clinical certifications were viewed as an aid to the establishment of safe and scientifically based exercise services within the framework of cardiac rehabilitation.

Over the last two decades, exercise has gained widespread favor as an important component in programs of rehabilitative care or health maintenance for an expanding list of chronic diseases and disabling conditions. The growth of public interest in the role of exercise in health promotion has been equally impressive. In addition, federal government policy makers have revisited questions of medical efficacy and financing for exercise services in rehabilitative care of selected CAD patients. Over the last several years, recommendations from the United States Public Health Service have increasingly acknowledged a central role for regular physical activity in the prevention of disease and promotion of health.

The development of the Health/Fitness Track certifications in the 1980's reflected ACSM's intent to increase the availability of qualified professionals to provide scientifically sound advice and supervision regarding appropriate physical activities for health maintenance in the apparently healthy adult population.

Since 1975, nearly 14,000 certificates have been awarded. With this growth, ACSM has taken steps to assure that its competency-based certifications will continue to be regarded as the premier program in the exercise field. A new periodical dealing with professional practice issues targeted to those who are certified, *ACSM Certified News*, is one example. Implementation of continuing education requirements for maintenance of certification is another. Continuing Education Credits can be accrued through ACSM-sponsored educational venues such as ACSM Workshops (Exercise Leader$_{SM}$, Health/Fitness Instructor$_{SM}$, Exercise Test Technologist$_{SM}$, and Exercise Specialist$_{SM}$), Regional Chapter and Annual Meetings, and other educational programs approved by the ACSM Professional Education Committee. These enhancements are intended to support continuing professional growth of those who have made a commitment to service in this rapidly growing health and fitness field. ACSM also acknowledges the expectation from successful candidates that the public will be informed of the high standards, values, and professionalism implicit in meeting these certification requirements. Most recently, the College has formally organized its volunteer committee structure and national office staff to give added emphasis to informing the public, professionals, and government agencies about issues of critical importance to ACSM. Informing these constituencies about the meaning and value of ACSM certification is one important priority that will be given attention in this new initiative.

ACSM CERTIFICATION PROGRAMS

The ACSM certifications are categorized by "tracks." The Health & Fitness Track is designed primarily for those individuals who provide leadership in programs of a preventive nature for apparently healthy individuals in corporate, commercial, or community settings. The Clinical Track is designed for those who may work with high-risk or diseased individuals as well as apparently healthy individuals.

Certification at a given level requires the candidate to have a knowledge and skill base commensurate with that specific level of certification. In addition, higher levels of certification incorporate the knowledge and skills associ-

CLINICAL TRACK			HEALTH/FITNESS TRACK		
Program Director (PD)	Exercise Specialist (ES)	Exercise Test Technologist (ETT)	Health/ Fitness Director (HFD)	Health/ Fitness Instructor (HFI)	Exercise Leader (EL)
PD	ES	ETT	HFD	HFI	EL
ES	ETT		HFI	EL	
ETT	HFI		EL		
HFD	EL				
HFI					
EL					

FIG. F–1. Each level of certification is responsible for the knowledge, skills, and abilities (KSAs) for all levels of certification listed below it, inclusive.

ated with other designated certification levels as illustrated by Figure F–1. Although there is no strict prerequisite experience or level of education required for taking certification examinations, each level of certification has been developed to include specific knowledge and skills at designated levels of employment. Professionals at these specified levels of employment would likely possess specific levels of academic training (including in some cases, graduate degrees) and experience. Therefore, recommendations for prerequisite education and experience are included for each level of certification.

For attaining and maintaining every level of ACSM certification, concurrent cardiopulmonary resuscitation (CPR) certification in basic life support (BLS) is a requirement.

HEALTH/FITNESS TRACK

There are three levels of certification within the Health/ Fitness Track:

Health/Fitness Director (HFD)®. The ACSM Health/Fitness Director ® is the highest level of certification in the Health/Fitness Track. Successful candidates must demonstrate administrative leadership skills for health and fitness programs in the corporate, commercial, or community setting primarily for apparently healthy individuals. Recommended training, experience, and attributes include:

- Educational training comparable to an undergraduate degree in a health and fitness curriculum or closely related field
- At least 1 year of experience in health and fitness program supervision
- The ability to organize and administer health and fitness programs
- A minimum of 3 years experience in an administrative management capacity of a health and fitness program

Health/Fitness Instructor (HFI)$_{SM}$. The ACSM Health/Fitness Instructor$_{SM}$ must demonstrate the ability to conduct exercise programs and provide health education for apparently healthy individuals. Recommended training, experience, and attributes include:

- Educational training comparable to an undergraduate or graduate degree in a health and fitness curriculum or closely related field
- Adequate knowledge of and skill in risk factor and health status identification, fitness appraisal, and exercise prescription
- Practical hands-on experience with exercise leadership
- Experience in lifestyle behavior modification counseling skills

Exercise Leader (EL)$_{SM}$. The ACSM Exercise Leader$_{SM}$ is the professional involved in "on-the-floor" exercise leadership. In addition to understanding basic physiological responses to exercise, the successful ACSM Exercise Leader$_{SM}$ must demonstrate "hands-on" techniques for teaching safe, effective, and fundamentally sound methods of exercise. Recommended training, experience, and attributes include:

- Practical experience with exercise leadership and instruction
- Ability to interact and communicate with others
- Ability to safely apply the principles of exercise and training to fitness programs
- Ability to answer basic questions related to exercise science and refer others to appropriate sources of information

---

CLINICAL TRACK

There are three levels of certification within the Clinical Track. For attaining and maintaining Clinical Track certification, concurrent CPR/BLS level C certification is a requirement.

Program Director (PD)$_{SM}$. ACSM Program Director$_{SM}$ is the highest level of certification in the Clinical Track. This certification is directed toward professionals whose primary responsibilities are developing and directing safe and effective clinical exercise programs. The ACSM PD$_{SM}$ certification requires a significant increase in breadth and depth of knowledge and experience beyond that of an Exercise Specialist$_{SM}$. Recommended training, experience, and attributes include:

- Post-baccalaureate degree or equivalent training in medicine or an allied health field plus 1 year of clinical experience
- Minimum of 1 year of recent experience in a position of administrative authority within a clinical exercise program
- Ability to organize and administer preventive and rehabilitative exercise programs

Exercise Specialist (ES)$_{SM}$. The successful ACSM Exercise Specialist$_{SM}$ candidate must demonstrate competence in graded exercise testing, exercise prescription, exercise leadership, patient counseling, and education in clinical exercise programs. Recommended training, experience, and attributes include:

- Minimum of 4 months/600 hours of practical experience in a clinical exercise program
- Baccalaureate degree in an allied health field or equivalent
- Ability to execute an accurate individualized prescription of activities for patients referred to clinical exercise programs
- Ability to effectively educate and/or counsel patients regarding activity and lifestyle issues

Exercise Test Technologist (ETT)$_{SM}$. The ACSM Exercise Test Technologist$_{SM}$ certification provides recognition for trained professionals who have demonstrated the knowledge, competence and skills necessary to deliver safe and valid exercise-related tests in a clinical health care environment. Recommended training, experience, and attributes include:

- Theoretical knowledge as applied to clinical graded exercise testing
- Ability to administer graded exercise testing procedures consistent with age and health status
- Competence in data recording, organization, and reporting
- Ability to effectively communicate and interact with patients
- Ability to Identify and implement appropriate emergency procedures

HOW TO OBTAIN INFORMATION AND APPLICATION MATERIALS

The certification programs of the American College of Sports Medicine are subject to continuous review and revision. Content development is entrusted to a committee of professional volunteers with expertise in science, medicine, and program management. Expertise in design and procedures for competency assessment is also represented on this committee. Administration of certification is the responsibility of the ACSM National Center. Inquiries concerning certifications, application requirements, fees, and examination test sites and dates may be made to:

> Director, Certification Department
> American College of Sports Medicine
> P.O. Box 1440
> Indianapolis, IN 46206-1440 USA

KNOWLEDGE, SKILLS, AND ABILITIES (KSAs) UNDERLYING ACSM CERTIFICATIONS

Minimal competencies for each certification level are outlined below. Certification examinations are constructed based upon these knowledges, skills and abilities (KSAs).

A companion ACSM publication, *Resource Manual for Guidelines for Exercise Testing and Prescription, 2nd ed.*, may be used to gain further insight pertaining to the topics identified here. It should be understood that neither the *Guidelines for Exercise Testing and Prescription* nor the *Resource Manual* provide all of the information upon which the ACSM Certification examinations are based. However, the *Resource Manual* may prove to be beneficial as a review of specific topics and as a general outline of many of the integral concepts to be mastered by those seeking certification.

As the level of certification increases, the depth of understanding and the knowledge base are expected to increase commensurately. Descriptive terms used in the KSAs have been selected to reflect the level of difficulty and to help define the extent of knowledge one must possess to successfully qualify for certification. For the first levels of certification, the verbs "define," "identify," and "list" have been used. The mid-level certification behavioral objectives use "describe," "calculate," "plot," and "demonstrate," which imply the candidate must be able to deal with the knowledge base on a more sophisticated level. Being able to describe, demonstrate, or mathematically manipulate principles, skills, or information reflects a greater understanding. The higher levels of certification demonstrate increasing complexity by using "discuss," "explain," "differentiate," "compare," and "teach." When the verb "discuss," "demonstrate," and "teach" are used, the candidate must be prepared to interact with another person, such as on a practical examination or with the physician, patient, or client in the workplace. Also, the candidate may be tested in written format with the understanding that the depth of knowledge and complexity of questions will be greater. Although the descriptive terms are generally stratified as described, they are not used exclusively at any level. For example, when appropriate, the descriptor "list" or "identify" may be used for one of the upper level behavioral objectives. Or, it may be equally appropriate to use "discuss" or "explain" at the lower level.

The KSAs are listed sequentially to demonstrate the concept that each higher level of certification is responsible for those KSAs listed under the certification in question, plus those listed under lower certification levels within a track. For example, a Health/Fitness Director® candidate is responsible for all KSAs that are listed under Health/Fitness Director,® Health/Fitness Instructor$_{SM}$ and Exercise Leader$_{SM}$ within each topic.

HEALTH/FITNESS TRACK CERTIFICATION KSAs

FUNCTIONAL ANATOMY AND BIOMECHANICS

EXERCISE LEADER_{SM}

1. Describe the basic structures of bone, skeletal muscle, and connective tissues.
2. Describe the basic anatomy of the heart, cardiovascular system, and respiratory system.
3. Identify the major bones and muscles and their actions. Major muscles include, but not limited to: trapezius, pectoralis major, latissiumus dorsi, biceps, triceps, abdominal, erector spinae, gluteus maximus, quadriceps, hamstrings, and gastrocnemius.
4. Define the following terms: supination, pronation, flexion, extension, adduction, abduction hyperextension, rotation, and circumduction.
5. List and describe the types of joints in the body.
6. Identify the interrelationships among center of gravity, base of support, balance, and stability.
7. Describe the following abnormal curvatures of the spine: lordosis, scoliosis, kyphosis.
8. Describe low back pain syndrome and describe exercises used to prevent this problem.
9. Describe the biomechanical effects and potential risks of using hand/ankle weights.

10. Describe and demonstrate exercises designed to enhance muscular strength and/or endurance of specific major muscle groups.
11. Describe and demonstrate exercises for enhancing musculoskeletal flexibility.

HEALTH/FITNESS INSTRUCTOR$_{SM}$

12. Describe the structure and nature of movement in the major joints of the body.
13. Describe the factors which determine range of motion in the major joints of the body.
14. Describe the biomechanical principles that underlie performance of the following activities: walking, jogging, running, swimming, cycling, weight lifting, and carrying or moving objects.
15. Locate the common sites for measurement of skinfold thickness, skeletal diameters, girth measurements for estimation of body composition; the anatomic landmarks for palpation of peripheral pulses; locate the brachial artery and correctly place the cuff and stethoscope in position of blood pressure measurement.

HEALTH/FITNESS DIRECTOR®

16. Discuss the relationship among biomechanical efficiency, oxygen cost of activity (economy), and performance of physical activity.
17. Discuss the application of biomechanical principles (e.g., Newton's Laws of Motion) to human movement.

EXERCISE PHYSIOLOGY

EXERCISE LEADER_{SM}

1. Define aerobic and anaerobic metabolism.
2. Identify the role of aerobic, anaerobic and ATP-PC systems in the performance of various physical activities.
3. Define the following terms: ischemia, angina pectoris, tachycardia, bradycardia, myocardial infarction, cardiac output, stroke volume, lactic acid, oxygen consumption, hyperventilation, systolic blood pressure, diastolic blood pressure.
4. Describe the role of carbohydrates, fats, proteins as fuels for aerobic and anaerobic metabolism.
5. Demonstrate an understanding of the components of fitness: cardiorespiratory fitness, muscular strength, muscular endurance, flexibility, body composition.
6. Define the major components of motor fitness: agility, speed, balance, coordination, power.
7. Describe the normal cardiorespiratory responses to static and dynamic exercise in terms of heart rate, blood pressure, and oxygen consumption.
8. Describe how heart rate, blood pressure, and oxygen consumption responses change with adaptation to chronic exercise training and how men and women may differ in response.
9. List the physiological adaptations associated with strength training in men and women.
10. Define and describe the relationship of METs and kilocalories to physical activity.
11. Identify the common sites for pulse palpation and describe how heart rate is determined by pulse palpation. List precautions in the application of these techniques.

12. Identify the physiological principles related to warm-up and cool-down.
13. List the effects of temperature, humidity, altitude, and pollution upon the physiological response to exercise.
14. Identify the physical and physiological signs of over-exercising, over-training, overuse.
15. Describe the common theories of muscle fatigue and delayed onset muscle soreness (DOMS).

HEALTH/FITNESS INSTRUCTOR_{SM}

16. Describe the primary anaerobic and aerobic energy systems and their role during exercise.
17. Describe the basic properties of cardiac muscle and the normal pathways of conduction in the heart.
18. Calculate the energy cost in METs and kilocalories for given exercise intensities in stepping exercise, bicycle ergometry, and during horizontal and graded walking and running.
19. Identify approximate MET equivalents for various sport, recreational, and work tasks.
20. Discuss the physiological basis of the major components of physical fitness: flexibility, cardiovascular fitness, muscular strength, muscular endurance, and body composition.
21. Explain the differences in the cardiorespiratory responses to static exercise compared with dynamic exercise, including possible hazards of static exercise.
22. Explain how the principle of specificity relates to the components of fitness.
23. Define and describe the implications of ventilatory anaerobic threshold ("anaerobic threshold") as it relates to physical conditioning programs and cardiovascular assessment.
24. Explain the concept of detraining or reversibility of conditioning and its implications in fitness programs.

25. Discuss the physical and psychological signs of over-training and provide recommendations to deal with these problems.

26. Describe the structure of the skeletal muscle fiber and the basic mechanism of contraction.

27. Describe the functional characteristics of fast and slow twitch fibers.

28. Explain contraction of muscle in terms of the sliding filament theory.

29. Explain twitch, summation, and tetanus in terms of muscle contraction.

30. Discuss the physiological principles involved in promoting gains in muscular strength and endurance.

31. Demonstrate an understanding of the relationship between number of repetitions, intensity, number of sets, and rest with regard to strength training.

32. Describe how each of the following differ from the normal condition: dyspnea, hypoxia, hypoventilation, orthostatic hypotension, premature atrial contractions, and premature ventricular contractions.

33. Describe blood pressure responses associated with exercise and changes in body position.

34. Define hypotension and hypertension and explain why blood pressure should be monitored during exercise testing.

35. List the physiologic adaptations to the muscular system, metabolism, and the cardiorespiratory system that occur at rest, during submaximal and maximal exercise following chronic anaerobic and aerobic training.

36. Describe the response of the following variables to steady state submaximal exercise and maximal exercise: heart rate, stroke volume, cardiac output, pulmonary ventilation, tidal volume, respiratory rate, arteriovenous oxygen difference.

37. Describe the physiologic and metabolic responses to

exercise associated with chronic disease (e.g., heart disease, hypertension, diabetes mellitus, and pulmonary disease).

HEALTH/FITNESS DIRECTOR®

38. Discuss the physiological and biochemical characteristics of fast and slow twitch muscle fibers.
39. Explain the concept of muscular fatigue during specific conditions of task, intensity, duration and the accumulative effects of exercise.
40. Contrast the cardiorespiratory responses to acute graded exercise in conditioned and unconditioned subjects.
41. Compare the relative and absolute cardiorespiratory responses to levels of exercise intensity in conditioned and unconditioned subjects.

HUMAN DEVELOPMENT AND AGING

EXERCISE LEADER

1. Describe the changes that occur in maturation from childhood to older adulthood for the following areas: skeletal muscle, bone structure, reaction and movement time, coordination, tolerance to hot and cold environments, maximal oxygen consumption, strength, flexibility, body composition, resting and maximal heart rate, resting and maximal blood pressure.
2. List the benefits and risks associated with exercise training in pre- and post-pubescent youth.
3. Identify benefits and precautions associated with resistance and endurance training in the older adult.
4. Describe special leadership techniques which might

be used for children, adolescents and older participants.

HEALTH/FITNESS INSTRUCTOR_{SM}

5. Demonstrate and understand the effect of the aging process on the structure and function of the human organism at rest, during exercise, and during recovery.
6. Characterize the differences in the development of an exercise prescription for children, adolescents, and older participants.
7. Describe the unique adaptations to exercise training in children, adolescents, and older participants with regard to strength, functional capacity, and motor skills.
8. Describe common orthopedic and cardiovascular considerations of older participants and what modifications in exercise prescription are indicated.

HEALTH/FITNESS DIRECTOR®

9. Demonstrate a knowledge and a practical understanding of programming techniques as they relate to markets of all ages.
10. Identify the various components involved with implementing successful programs for children, adolescents, adults, and older participants.

PATHOPHYSIOLOGY/RISK FACTORS

EXERCISE LEADER_{SM}

1. Identify risk factors for coronary artery disease (CAD) and designate those that may be favorably modified by regular and appropriate physical activity habits.

2. Define the following terms: total cholesterol, high density lipoprotein cholesterol (HDL-C), low density lipoprotein cholesterol (LDL-C), total cholesterol/high density lipoprotein cholesterol ratio, anemia, and hypertension.

3. Be familiar with the plasma cholesterol levels for various ages as recommended by the National Cholesterol Education Program.

4. Identify the following cardiovascular risk factors or conditions which may require consultation with medical or allied health professionals prior to participation in physical activity or prior to a major increase in physical activity intensities and habits: inappropriate resting; exercise and recovery HR's and BP's; new discomfort or changes in the pattern of discomfort in the chest area, neck, shoulder or arm with exercise or at rest; heart murmurs; myocardial infarction; fainting or dizzy spells, claudication, ischemia, cigarette or other tobacco use, lipoprotein profile.

5. Identify the following respiratory risk factors which may require consultation with medical professionals prior to participation in physical activity or prior to major increases in physical activities or habits; extreme breathlessness after mild exertion or during sleep, asthma, exercise-induced asthma, bronchitis, emphysema.

6. Identify the following metabolic risk factors that may require consultation with medical professionals prior to participation in physical activity or prior to major increases in physical activity intensities and habits: body weight more than 20% above optimal, thyroid disease, diabetes or glucose intolerance, McArdle's syndrome, hypoglycemia.

7. Identify the following musculoskeletal risk factors which may require consultation with medical profes-

sionals prior to physical activity or prior to major increases in physical activity intensities and habits: osteoarthritis, rheumatoid arthritis, acute or chronic back pain, prosthesis-artificial joints.

8. Demonstrate an understanding of muscle atrophy and the loss of strength and endurance with disuse/sedentary behavior.

9. Define shin splints, sprains, strains, tennis elbow, bursitis, stress fracture, tendinitis, contusions, osteoporosis, arthritis, overweight, chondromalacia, blisters, skin irritations and low back discomfort.

HEALTH/FITNESS INSTRUCTOR$_{SM}$

10. Demonstrate an understanding of the pathophysiology of atherosclerosis and how this process is influenced by physical activity.

11. Identify common drugs from each of the following classes of medications and describe the principal action and the effects on exercise testing and prescription:
    A. Antianginal (nitrates, beta blockers, calcium channel blockers, etc.)
    B. Antihypertensive
    C. Antiarrhythmic
    D. Bronchodilators
    E. Hypoglycemics
    F. Psychotropics
    G. Vasodilators

12. Identify the effects of the following substances on exercise responses: antihistamines, tranquilizers, alcohol, diet pills, cold tablets, caffeine, and nicotine.

HEALTH/FITNESS DIRECTOR®

13. Explain the risk factor concept of coronary artery disease (CAD) and the influence of heredity and lifestyle upon the development of CAD.
14. Explain the process of atherosclerosis, the factors involved in its genesis, and the methods which may potentially reverse the process.
15. Discuss in detail how lifestyle factors and heredity influence lipid and lipoprotein profiles.
16. Explain the genesis of myocardial ischemia and infarction.
17. Explain the causes of hypertension, obesity, hyperlipidemia, diabetes, chronic obstructive and restrictive pulmonary diseases, arthritis, and gout.
18. Identify and explain the effects of the above diseases or conditions on cardiorespiratory and metabolic function at rest and during exercise.
19. Describe muscular, cardiorespiratory, and metabolic responses to exercise following a decrease in physical activity, bed rest, or casting of a limb for a period of one month.
20. Identify and discuss the causes and mechanisms of chronic obstructive pulmonary disease (COPD), exercise-induced asthma, chronic asthma, chronic diseases, and immunosuppressive disease.
21. Identify current drugs from each of the following classes of medications. Explain the principal action, mechanism of action, and major side-effects.
    A. Antianginal
    B. Antihypertensive
    C. Antiarrhythmic
    D. Bronchodilators
    E. Hypoglycemics
    F. Psychotropics
    G. Vasodilators

HUMAN BEHAVIOR/PSYCHOLOGY

EXERCISE LEADER_{SM}

1. List several techniques to deal with disruptive individuals in group programs (e.g., non-complier, comedian, chronic complainer, and the over-exerciser)
2. Define the psychological principles which are critical to health behavior change (i.e., behavior modification, reinforcement, goal-setting, social support and peer pressure.)
3. Describe the personal communication skills necessary to develop rapport in order to motivate individuals to begin exercise, enhance adherence, and return to exercise.
4. Identify several techniques which can be used in an exercise program to facilitate skill development in muscular relaxation.
5. List specific techniques to enhance motivation: posters, recognition, bulletin boards, games, competitions, etc.

HEALTH/FITNESS INSTRUCTOR_{SM}

6. Describe the specific strategies (e.g., operant conditioning) aimed at encouraging the initiation, adherence, and return to participation in an exercise program or any other healthy lifestyle behaviors.
7. Describe effective counseling communication skills in order to bring about behavioral change.
8. Describe how each of the following terms may impact upon the successful management of an exercise program: anxiety, depression, fear, denial, rejection, rationalization, aggression, anger, hostility, empathy, arousal, euphoria, and relaxation.

9. Discuss the potential manifestation of test anxiety (i.e., performance, appraisal threat) during exercise testing and how it may disrupt accurate physiological responses to testing.

10. Describe the differential effects of exercise and progressive relaxation as stress management techniques for modifying anxiety, depression, anger, and for generating relaxation.

11. Discuss the behavioral change strategies which are appropriate or inappropriate for modifying body composition.

HEALTH/FITNESS DIRECTOR®

12. Describe basic cognitive-behavioral intervention such as shaping, goal-setting, motivation, cueing, problem solving, reinforcement strategies, and relaxation management.

13. Describe the selection of appropriate behavioral and outcome goals, and the suggested method and frequency of outcome evaluation.

HEALTH APPRAISAL AND FITNESS TESTING

EXERCISE LEADER_{SM}

1. Describe and demonstrate the use of health history appraisal to obtain information on past and present medical history, orthopedic limitations, prescribed medications, activity patterns, nutritional habits, stress and anxiety levels, family history of heart disease, smoking history, and use of alcohol and illicit drugs and know when to recommend medical clearance.

2. Describe the use of informed consent forms and medical clearances prior to exercise participation.
3. Demonstrate the ability to conduct group field assessments such as Cooper 12-minute test, step test, strength, muscular endurance, and flexibility assessment.
4. State the rationale for determining body composition.
5. Describe the types of tests for cardiorespiratory fitness, evaluation of strength and flexibility, and techniques used to determine body composition and the purposes for which each may be used (i.e., base-line, comparison, motivation, etc.)
6. Describe the difference between maximal and submaximal cardiorespiratory exercise tests.
7. Demonstrate the ability to measure pulse rate accurately both at rest and during exercise.
8. Demonstrate the ability to measure blood pressure accurately at rest.

HEALTH/FITNESS INSTRUCTOR$_{SM}$

9. Demonstrate or identify appropriate techniques for health appraisal and use of fitness evaluations.
10. State the purpose and demonstrate basic principles of exercise testing.
11. Describe the categories of participants who should receive medical clearance prior to administration of an exercise test or participation in an exercise program.
12. Identify relative and absolute contraindications to exercise testing or participation.
13. Demonstrate the ability to obtain appropriate medical history, informed consent, and other pertinent information prior to exercise testing.
14. Discuss the limitations of informed consent and medical clearances prior to exercise testing.

15. Demonstrate the ability to instruct participants in the use of equipment and test procedures.
16. Demonstrate the ability to assess muscular strength, muscular endurance, and flexibility.
17. Demonstrate various techniques of assessing body composition and discuss the advantages/disadvantages and limitations of the various techniques.
18. Discuss and demonstrate various submaximal and maximal cardiorespiratory fitness tests using various modes of exercise and interpret and critique the information obtained from the various tests.
19. Discuss modification of protocols and procedures for cardiorespiratory fitness tests in children, adolescents, and older adults.
20. Explain the purpose and procedures for monitoring clients prior to, during, and after cardiorespiratory fitness testing.
21. Demonstrate the ability to accurately measure heart rate, blood pressure, and rating of perceived exertion at rest and during exercise according to established guidelines.
22. Demonstrate the ability to interpret results of fitness evaluations on apparently healthy individuals and those with stable disease.
23. Describe and demonstrate techniques for calibration of a cycle ergometer and a motor-driven treadmill.
24. Identify appropriate criteria for discontinuing a fitness evaluation and demonstrate proper procedures to be followed after discontinuing such a test.

HEALTH/FITNESS DIRECTOR®

25. Explain the use and value of the results of the exercise test and fitness evaluation for various populations.

26. Demonstrate the ability to design and implement a health appraisal/fitness assessment programming; including but not limited to staffing needs, physician interaction, documents, equipment, marketing, ongoing evaluations.
27. Demonstrate the ability to recruit, train and evaluate appropriate staff personnel for performing exercise tests and fitness evaluations.

EMERGENCY PROCEDURES AND SAFETY

EXERCISE LEADER$_{SM}$

1. Demonstrate skills necessary to obtain basic life support and cardiopulmonary resuscitation certification.
2. Describe appropriate emergency procedures (i.e., telephone procedures, written emergency procedures, personnel responsibilities, etc.) in a variety of exercise settings.
3. Describe basic first aid procedures for exercise-related injuries such as: bleeding skin wounds, contusions, strains/sprains, fractures, dizziness, syncope and metabolic abnormalities including hypo/hypertension, hypo/hyperglycemia, hypo/hyperthermia.
4. Demonstrate an understanding of the risks associated with exercise participation.
5. Describe the signs/symptoms for participants (including special populations) to defer, delay, or terminate the exercise session.
6. Demonstrate the basic precautions taken in a weight room area to ensure participant safety (e.g., spotting, buddy system, control speed of movement, weights returned to rack, safe passageways, check loose parts on equipment, etc.)

HEALTH/FITNESS INSTRUCTOR_{SM}

7. Demonstrate knowledge of safety plans, emergency procedures, and first aid techniques needed during fitness evaluations, exercise testing, and exercise training.
8. Identify the components that create and maintain a safe environment.
9. Identify the content and discuss the use of informed consent and exercise waivers.
10. Discuss the instructors responsibilities, limitations, and the legal implications of carrying out emergency procedures.
11. Describe potential musculoskeletal injuries (e.g., contusions, strains/sprains, fractures), cardiovascular/pulmonary complications (e.g., tachycardia, bradycardia, hypo/hypertension, tachypnea), and metabolic abnormalities (e.g., fainting/syncope, hypo/hyperglycemia, hypo/hyperthermia).
12. Explain the initial management and first aid techniques associated with open wounds, musculoskeletal injuries, cardiovascular/pulmonary complications, and metabolic abnormalities.
13. Describe the components of an equipment maintenance/repair program and how it may be used to evaluate the condition of exercise equipment in order to reduce potential risk of injury.

HEALTH/FITNESS DIRECTOR®

14. Provide instruction in the principles and techniques used in cardiopulmonary resuscitation.
15. Design and update emergency procedures for a preventive exercise program and an exercise testing facility.
16. List emergency drugs which should be available during exercise testing.

17. Train staff in safety procedures, the epidemiology of risk of injury and cardiovascular complications, risk reduction techniques, and emergency techniques.
18. Demonstrate an understanding of the legal implications of documented safety procedures, the use of incident documents, ongoing training, and drills.

EXERCISE PROGRAMMING

EXERCISE LEADER_{SM}

1. State the recommended intensity, duration, frequency, and type of physical activity necessary for development of cardiorespiratory fitness in an apparently healthy population.
2. Differentiate between the dose of exercise required for various health benefits and that required for fitness development.
3. Describe the differences between improvement and maintenance exercise training programs.
4. Describe the principles of overload, specificity and progression and how they relate to exercise programming.
5. Describe and demonstrate appropriate exercises used in warm-up and cool-down for: cardiorespiratory conditioning classes, weight training and sport participation (racquet sports, volleyball, basketball, etc.).
6. Demonstrate an understanding for the components incorporated into an exercise session and their proper sequence (i.e., warm-up, aerobic stimulus phase, cool-down, muscular endurance and flexibility).
7. Define overload, specificity of exercise conditioning, use-disuse, progressive resistance, isotonic, isometric, isokinetic, concentric, eccentric, atrophy, hypertrophy, sets, repetitions, plyometrics, Valsalva maneuver.

8. Define RPE and describe the relationship to the physiologic responses to exercise and its role in exercise programming.

9. Demonstrate an understanding of calculation of predicted maximal and training heart rate ranges.

10. Demonstrate various methods for monitoring exercise intensity such as heart rate and perceived exertion.

11. Describe the signs and symptoms of excessive effort which would indicate a change in intensity, duration, or frequency of exercise.

12. Describe and demonstrate appropriate modifications in exercise programs which may be recommended by a physician for the following: older adults, acute illness, controlled conditions such as exercise-induced asthma, allergies, hypertension, pregnancy and postpartum, obesity, and low back pain.

13. Demonstrate the ability to recognize proper technique and use of all exercise equipment (i.e., proper body mechanics, proper positioning on apparatus, appropriate settings for cardiovascular and resistance training, proper monitoring techniques, safety considerations, etc.).

14. Describe the importance of flexibility and recommend proper exercises for improving range of motion of all major joints.

15. Demonstrate the ability to modify exercises in the group setting for apparently healthy persons of various fitness levels.

16. Describe and demonstrate exercises for the improvement and maintenance of muscular endurance and muscular strength.

17. Describe how the following weight training methods may be used in resistance programming: progressive resistance exercise, super sets, pyramiding, split routines, plyometrics, isokinetic, isotonic, isometric.

18. Identify various types of isometric, isotonic, and isokinetic equipment.

19. List advantages and disadvantages of various aerobic exercise equipment such as stair climbers, rowing machines, treadmills, bicycles, etc.

20. Describe the hypothetical concerns and potential risks which may be associated with the use of exercises such as straight leg sit-ups, double leg raises, full squats, hurdler's stretch, plough, forceful back hyperextension, and standing straight leg toe touch.

21. Describe the differences between interval, continuous and circuit training programs.

22. Demonstrate appropriate and effective group exercise management and teaching techniques

23. Describe various locations a leader may take within a group to enhance visibility, participant interactions, and communication.

24. Demonstrate the ability to communicate effectively with exercise participants in the group and one-on-one setting.

25. Describe an exercise regimen for a water exercise class.

26. Describe partner resistance exercises which can be employed in a class setting.

27. Demonstrate a knowledge of techniques for accommodating various fitness levels within the same class.

28. Identify the differences between high impact and low impact exercise classes and which class is appropriate for various participants.

29. Identify the short-term and long-range advantages/benefits associated with fitness participation.

HEALTH/FITNESS INSTRUCTOR$_{SM}$

30. Design, implement, and evaluate individualized and group exercise programs based on health history and physical fitness assessments.

31. Define exercise prescription guidelines for apparently healthy, higher risk, and clients with controlled disease.

32. Demonstrate the use of the variables of mode, intensity, duration, frequency, and progression in designing cardiorespiratory and resistive training.
33. Design exercise programs to improve or maintain cardiorespiratory endurance.
34. Demonstrate the use of various methods for establishing and monitoring levels of exercise intensity including heart rate, RPE, and METs.
35. Design resistive exercise programs to increase or maintain muscular strength and/or endurance for the purpose of general fitness, hypertrophy, injury prevention, and sports conditioning.
36. Demonstrate the proper techniques for performing resistive exercises for all major muscle groups using calisthenics, free weights, resistive equipment and machines.
37. Demonstrate an ability to establish appropriate resistance levels on circuit weight training equipment and various free weight exercises.
38. Design flexibility programs to improve or maintain range of motion at all major joints.
39. Demonstrate proper techniques for performing flexibility exercises for all major muscle groups.
40. Discuss the advantages and disadvantages of implementation of interval, continuous, and circuit training programs, and design programs for each.
41. Discuss the advantages and disadvantages of various commercial exercise equipment in developing cardiorespiratory fitness, muscular strength, and muscular endurance.
42. Describe special precautions and modifications of exercise programming for participation at altitude, different ambient temperatures, humidities, and environmental pollution.
43. Describe modifications in type, duration, frequency, progression level of supervision, and monitoring tech-

niques in exercise programs for patients with heart disease, diabetes mellitus, obesity, hypertension, musculoskeletal problems, pregnancy/postpartum, and exercise-induced asthma.

44. Demonstrate an understanding for the components incorporated into an exercise session and their proper sequence (i.e., pre-exercise evaluation, warm-up, aerobic stimulus phase, cool-down, muscular endurance, and flexibility).

45. Describe the types of exercise programs available in the community and how these programs are appropriate for various populations.

46. Demonstrate an understanding of the importance of recording exercise sessions and performing periodic evaluations to assess changes in fitness status.

NUTRITION AND WEIGHT MANAGEMENT

EXERCISE LEADER$_{SM}$

1. Define the following terms: obesity, overweight, percent fat, lean body mass, anorexia nervosa, bulimia, and body fat distribution.

2. Discuss the relationship between body composition and health.

3. Compare the effects of diet plus exercise, diet alone, and exercise alone as methods for modifying body composition.

4. Describe misconceptions about spot reductions and rapid weight loss programs.

5. Explain the concept of energy balance as it relates to weight control.

6. Identify the functions of fat and water soluble vitamins and contrast their potential risk of toxicity with over-supplementation.

7. Discuss the ramifications of the use of salt tablets, diet pills, protein powder, and other nutritional supplements.

8. Describe the importance of and procedures for maintaining normal hydration at times of heavy sweating, and describe appropriate beverages for fluid replacement during and after exercise.

9. Demonstrate familiarity with the USDA Food Pyramid and US Dietary Guidelines.

10. Demonstrate an understanding of the importance of calcium and iron in women's health.

11. Describe the effects of diet and exercise on the blood lipid profile.

12. Describe the myths and consequences associated with inappropriate weight loss methods: saunas, vibrating belts, body wraps, electric simulators and sweat suits.

13. List the number of kilocalories in one gram of the following: fat, carbohydrate, protein, and alcohol. List the number of kilocalories in one pound of fat.

14. Describe appropriate weekly weight loss goals.

HEALTH/FITNESS INSTRUCTOR$_{SM}$

15. List the six essential nutrients and describe their nutritional role.

16. Discuss the recommended distribution of calories from fat, carbohydrate, and protein.

17. Describe the health implications of variation in body fat distribution patterns and the significance of waist/hip ratios.

18. Discuss guidelines for caloric intake for an individual desiring to lose or gain weight.

19. Discuss common nutritional ergogenic aids, their purported mechanism of action and any risks and/or benefits (e.g., carbohydrate, protein/amino acids, vitamins, minerals, sodium bicarbonate, bee pollen, etc.).

20. Describe nutritional factors related to the female athlete triad syndrome (i.e., eating disorders, menstrual cycle abnormalities, and osteopetrosis).

21. Demonstrate familiarity with the NIH Consensus statement of health risks of obesity, Nutrition for Physical Fitness Position Paper of the American Dietetic Association (endorsed by ACSM), and the ACSM Position Stand on proper and improper weight loss programs.

PROGRAM ADMINISTRATION/ MANAGEMENT

HEALTH/FITNESS INSTRUCTOR_{SM}

1. Understand the health fitness instructor's supportive role in administration and program management within a health/fitness facility.

2. Demonstrate an ability to administer fitness-related programs within established budgetary guidelines.

3. Demonstrate an ability to develop marketing materials for the purpose of promoting fitness-related programs.

4. Describe various sales techniques for prospective program clients/participants.

5. Describe the documentation required when a client shows signs or symptoms during an exercise session which should be referred to a physician.

6. Demonstrate the ability to create and maintain records pertaining to participant exercise adherence, retention, and goal setting.

7. Demonstrate the ability to develop and administer educational programs (i.e., lectures, workshops, etc.) and educational materials (i.e., participant handouts).

8. Demonstrate an understanding of management of a fitness department (e.g., working with a budget,

training exercise leaders, scheduling, running staff
meetings, etc.).

9. Discuss the importance of tracking and evaluating
member retention.

HEALTH/FITNESS DIRECTOR®

10. Describe a management plan for the development of
staff, materials for education, marketing, client
records, billing, facilities management, and financial
planning.
11. Discuss how each of the following affect the decision-
making process: budget, market analysis, program
evaluation, facilities, staff allocation, and community
development.
12. Discuss the development, evaluation, and revision of
policies and procedures for programming, and elements of a program evaluation report.
13. Discuss the use of outside consultation: establishing
contacts, contracting for services and follow-up procedures.
14. Discuss how the computer can assist in data analysis,
spreadsheet development, and daily tracking of customer service and utilization.
15. Describe and discuss the management-by-objective
decision-making approach.
16. Interpret applied research in the areas of testing, exercise, and educational programs in order to maintain a
comprehensive and current state-of-the-art program.
17. Compare and contrast the various evaluation design
models such as cross-sectional, longitudinal, case
control, and randomized clinical trials.
18. Discuss the establishment of a database, including
type of data to be collected, data management and
analysis.
19. Discuss the organization of a risk factor screening pro-

gram; describe procedures, staff training, feedback, and follow-up.

Personnel

20. Demonstrate an understanding of personnel management.
21. Describe effective interviewing, hiring, and employee termination procedures.
22. Diagram and explain an organizational chart and show the staff relationships between a health fitness director, governing body, medical advisor, and staff.
23. Discuss various staff training techniques.
24. Describe performance reviews and their role in evaluating staff.
25. Discuss legal obligations and problems involved in personnel management.
26. Discuss incentive-based compensation management.
27. Describe effective methods of implementing a sales commission system.
28. Discuss the significance of a benefits program for staff.
29. Describe the process of establishing a wage-based scale.
30. Identify the procedures of writing and implementing job descriptions.
31. Describe personnel time management techniques.

Budget/Finance

32. Demonstrate an understanding of the principles of financial management.
33. Demonstrate an understanding of basic accounting principles such as accounts payable, accounts receivable, liabilities, assets, and return on investment.
34. Identify the various forms of a business enterprise such as sole proprietorship, partnership, corporation and S-corporation.
35. Identify the procedures involved with developing,

evaluating, revising, and updating capital and operating budgets.

36. Describe recommended expense management techniques.
37. Develop an understanding of taxes and how they impact various health/fitness organizations.
38. Develop an understanding of financial statement analysis.
39. Demonstrate an understanding of the current financial industry trends.
40. Demonstrate an understanding of program-related break-even analysis.
41. Discuss the importance of return on investment.
42. Demonstrate an understanding of the principles of operational costs versus revenue generated in regard to membership programs and profit centers.

Marketing/Sales

43. Demonstrate an understanding of sales and marketing.
44. Identify the steps in the development, implementation, and evaluation of a marketing plan.
45. Discuss the components of a needs assessment/market analysis.
46. Describe the various sales techniques for prospective members.
47. Discuss techniques for advertising, marketing, sales promotion, and public relations.
48. Discuss the principles of evaluating product and establishing pricing.
49. Describe various membership tracking techniques and the steps of implementation and evaluation of a plan.

Operations

50. Demonstrate an understanding for implementing capital improvements.

51. Discuss the principles of pricing and purchasing equipment and supplies.
52. Demonstrate an understanding of facility layout and design.
53. Demonstrate the ability to establish and evaluate an equipment preventive maintenance and repair program.
54. Describe a plan for implementing a daytime and nighttime housekeeping program.
55. Describe the importance of short-term and long-term planning.
56. Identify and explain operating policies for preventive exercise programs including data analysis and reporting, reimbursement of service fees, confidentiality of records, relationships between program and referring physicians, continuing education of participants and family, legal liability, and accident or injury reporting.
57. Explain the legal concepts of tort, negligence, contributory negligence, liability, indemnification, standards of care, consent, contract, confidentiality, malpractice, and the legal concerns regarding emergency procedures and informed consent.

Member Service/Communication

58. Demonstrate effective skills and techniques for communication and public speaking.
59. Discuss various techniques for obtaining customer feedback.
60. Describe an understanding of developing surveys for the purpose of customer communication.
61. Discuss the strategies for managing conflict.
62. Identify the recommended techniques of effective front desk management.

HEALTH PROMOTION

HEALTH/FITNESS DIRECTOR®

1. Demonstrate an understanding of health promotion programs, such as nutrition and weight management, smoking cessation, stress management, healthy back, substance abuse, and dependent care.
2. Discuss appropriate content within specific health promotion programs.
3. Discuss different methods utilized in implementing health promotion programs (e.g., health communications, referral programs, sponsored intervention programs, etc.).
4. Discuss resources available for various programs and delivery systems.
5. Discuss appropriate selection criteria for programs and providers.
6. Demonstrate an understanding of the role of evaluating health promotion programs in reducing health care costs and improving profitability in the work place.
7. Describe the concepts of cost-effectiveness and cost-benefit as it relates to the evaluation of health promotion programming in the workplace.
8. Discuss the means and amounts by which health promotion programs might reduce health care costs and improve profitability in the workplace.
9. Demonstrate an understanding of how health promotion programs may interrelate with Employee Assistance Programs (EAPs).

CLINICAL TRACK
CERTIFICATION KSAs

FUNCTIONAL ANATOMY AND BIOMECHANICS

EXERCISE TEST TECHNOLOGIST_{SM}

1. Demonstrate a knowledge of surface anatomy as related to exercise testing and fitness evaluation.
2. Locate the appropriate sites for the limb and chest leads for standard and bipolar resting and exercise ECGs.
3. Locate the brachial artery and describe the cuff and stethoscope positions for blood pressure measurement.
4. Locate anatomic landmarks for palpation of radial, brachial, and carotid pulses.
5. Locate the anatomic landmarks used during cardiopulmonary resuscitation and emergency defibrillation.

EXERCISE SPECIALIST_{SM}

6. Demonstrate an understanding of the biomechanical factors associated with various disease states, neuromuscular disorders, and orthopedic problems.
7. Discuss common gait abnormalities.
8. Discuss abnormal curvatures of the spine and their effects on the biomechanics of movement.
9. Discuss how muscular weakness and/or neurologic disorder affect the biomechanics of movement.

10. Locate common sites for measurement of skinfold thicknesses, widths, and girths.

EXERCISE PHYSIOLOGY

EXERCISE TEST TECHNOLOGIST$_{SM}$

1. Demonstrate a knowledge of exercise physiology as it relates to exercise testing.
2. List the cardiorespiratory responses associated with postural changes.
3. List the differences in the physiological responses to various modes ergometry, i.e., treadmill, cycle, or arm ergometer as they relate to exercise testing.
4. Describe the principle of specificity of training as it relates to the mode of exercise testing.
5. Explain the meaning of maximal oxygen (O_2) consumption and how it is measured.
6. Describe the normal cardiorespiratory responses to graded exercise.
7. Explain the common variables measured during cardiopulmonary exercise testing including heart rate slope, anaerobic threshold, ventilatory slope, maximum ventilation, breathing pattern, wasted ventilation, and wasted pulmonary circulation and their relationship to various diseases.

EXERCISE SPECIALIST$_{SM}$

8. Demonstrate an understanding of clinical applications of exercise physiology.
9. Describe the aerobic and anaerobic metabolic demands of various exercises for patients with cardiovascular, pulmonary, and/or metabolic diseases undergoing rehabilitation and their implications.

10. Describe how each of the following varies for the healthy individual vs. the patient with coronary artery disease (CAD): function of the myocardium, the generation of the action potential, repolarization, and major variants in pathways of electrical activity.

11. Describe the cardiovascular responses to postural change before and after exercise testing.

12. List and be able to plot the normal resting and exercise values associated with increasing exercise intensity (and how they may differ from the CAD and/or COPD patient) for: heart rate, stroke volume, cardiac output, double product, arteriovenous O_2 difference, O_2 consumption, systolic and diastolic blood pressure, minute ventilation, tidal volume, and breathing frequency.

13. Discuss the potential hazards of isometric exercise for subjects with low functional capacity or patients with cardiovascular disease.

14. Describe the physiological effects of bed rest and discuss the appropriate physical activities which might be used to counteract these changes.

15. Compare the unique hemodynamic responses of arm vs. leg exercise and of static vs. dynamic exercise.

16. Identify activities which are primarily aerobic or anaerobic.

17. Describe the determinants of myocardial O_2 consumption and the effects of exercise training on those determinants.

PROGRAM DIRECTOR$_{SM}$

18. Discuss the mechanisms by which functional capacity and cardiovascular, respiratory metabolic, endocrine, and neuromuscular adaptations occur in response to physical conditioning programs.

HUMAN DEVELOPMENT AND AGING

EXERCISE TEST TECHNOLOGIST_{SM}

1. Demonstrate competence in selecting an appropriate test protocol according to the age of the patient.
2. Describe adjustments which may be necessary for testing younger and older patients; specifically, instructions to the patient and modification of the testing protocol and equipment.

PROGRAM DIRECTOR_{SM}

3. Explain differences in overall policy and procedures for the inclusion of different age groups in an exercise program.
4. Discuss facility and equipment adaptations necessary for different age groups.

HUMAN BEHAVIOR AND PSYCHOLOGY

EXERCISE TEST TECHNOLOGIST_{SM}

1. Demonstrate knowledge of psychological factors which may affect exercise test patients.
2. Identify factors which may increase anxiety in the patient undergoing exercise testing and describe how anxiety in a patient may be reduced.
3. Identify specific psychological and physiological manifestations of test anxiety which can influence the response to an exercise test.

EXERCISE SPECIALIST$_{SM}$

4. Demonstrate an understanding of basic behavioral psychology and group dynamics as they apply to crisis management, coping, and lifestyle modifications.
5. Describe signs and symptoms of maladjustment/failure to cope during an illness crisis and/or personal adjustment crisis (e.g., job loss) that might prompt a psychological consult or referral to other professional services.
6. Describe the general principles of crisis management and factors influencing coping and learning in illness states.
7. Describe the psychological issues to be confronted by the patient and by family members of patients who have cardiorespiratory disease, and/or who have had an acute MI or cardiac surgery.
8. Contrast the psychological issues associated with an acute cardiac event vs. those associated with chronic cardiac conditions.
9. Describe the psychological stages involved with the acceptance of death and dying and recognize when it is necessary for a psychological consult or referral to a professional resource available in the community.

PROGRAM DIRECTOR$_{SM}$

10. Demonstrate an understanding of the need for psychosocial consultation and referral of individuals who exhibit signs of psychological distress.
11. Describe community resources for psychosocial support and behavior modification and outline an example of a referral system.
12. Describe the observable signs and symptoms of psychological distress secondary to cardiopulmonary disorders.

PATHOPHYSIOLOGY AND RISK FACTORS

EXERCISE TEST TECHNOLOGIST_{SM}

1. Demonstrate knowledge of the basic pathophysiology of coronary artery and pulmonary dieases.
2. Define myocardial ischemia and list the methods that are used to measure ischemic responses.
3. List the effects of CAD (including MI) upon performance and safety during an exercise test.
4. List primary and secondary risk factors for CAD.
5. Describe abnormal chronotropic and inotropic responses to exercise testing.
6. Explain indications for combining exercise testing with radionuclide imaging.
7. Describe common procedures used for radionuclide imaging (such as thallium, technetium, sestamibi, SPECT, RVG, MUGA, etc.).
8. Name the drugs commonly encountered during exercise testing and describe how they may affect the ECG, heart rate, or blood pressure at rest or during exercise (see Appendix A).
   A. Cardiovascular agents (beta adrenergic blockers, nitrates, calcium channel antagonists, antiarrhythmics, ACE-inhibitors)
   B. Anticoagulant and antiplatelet drugs (dipyridamole, aspirin, etc.)
   C. Digitalis glycosides
   D. Decongestants and antihistamines
   E. Diabetes agents (oral and injection)
   F. Electrolytes (potassium, etc.)
   G. Hormones (estrogen, thyroid preparations, etc.)
   H. Lipid-lowering agents.
   I. Psychotropic agents (antianxiety, antidepressants, antipsychotic agents, etc.)
   J. Respiratory therapy agents (bronchial dilators)

   K. Seizure disorders

   L. Smoking cessation aids (nicotine gum, nicotine patches, etc.)

9. Define reversible airway (obstructive) and restrictive lung diseases and how they may affect exercise testing.

EXERCISE SPECIALIST$_{SM}$

10. Demonstrate an understanding of the cardiorespiratory and metabolic responses to increasing intensities of exercise in certain diseases and conditions.

11. Describe the cardiorespiratory and metabolic responses in myocardial dysfunction and ischemia at rest and during exercise.

12. Describe the cardiorespiratory and metabolic responses which accompany or result from pulmonary diseases at rest and during exercise.

13. Describe the signs and symptoms of peripheral vascular diseases and the effects different types of exercise may have on each.

14. Describe the metabolic responses and possible complications of a diabetic patient at rest and during exercise.

15. Describe the influence of exercise on weight reduction, hyperlipidemia, and diabetes.

16. Describe the effects of variation in ambient temperature, humidity, CO_2, and altitude on functional capacity and the exercise prescription. Explain required adaptations to the exercise prescription when environmental extremes exist.

17. Describe the etiology of atherosclerosis.

18. Describe the implications, symptoms, and mechanisms of classical and vasospastic angina.

19. Describe the methods used to measure ischemic responses.

20. Discuss the pathophysiology of the healing myocardium and the potential complications which may occur after an acute MI (extension, expansion, rupture, etc.)

21. Discus *Risk Stratification* of patients after MI. What materials are used and what are the prognostic indicators for high risk patients post MI?

22. Describe the effects of the following classifications of drugs on the ECG, heart rate, and blood pressure. Also, list the common major symptoms of drug intolerance or toxicity in the following classes of medications (see Appendix A).

    A. Antianginal (nitrates, beta adrenergic blockers, calcium channel antagonists, etc.)
    B. Antiarrhythmic
    C. Anticoagulant and antiplatelet
    D. Lipid-lowering drugs
    E. Antihypertensive (diuretics, vasodilators, etc.)
    F. Digitalis glycosides
    G. Bronchodilators
    H. Tranquilizers, antidepressants, and antianxiety drugs
    I. Hypoglycemics

23. List the major effects of the above eleven classes of drugs on physiologic responses and symptomatology, including ECG changes, at rest and during exercise testing and training.

24. Demonstrate an understanding of various modalities applied in the medical diagnosis and therapeutic management of certain diseases.

25. Describe the purpose and utility of coronary angiography and radionuclide imaging.

26. Describe percutaneous transluminal coronary angioplasty (PTCA).

27. Describe the use of streptokinase and other thrombolytic agents.

PROGRAM DIRECTOR$_{SM}$

28. Demonstrate an understanding of the relationship between different disease states and rehabilitative therapy.
29. Explain the process of atherosclerosis including current hypotheses regarding onset and rate of progression and/or regression.
30. Demonstrate an understanding of lipoprotein classifications and their relationship to atherosclerosis or other diseases.
31. Contrast the signs and symptoms in the pulmonary vs. cardiac patient during exercise testing and exercise training.
32. Explain the diagnostic and prognostic value of the results of the graded exercise test for various populations.
33. Explain the diagnostic and prognostic value of the low level predischarge exercise test vs. the symptom-limited test and the indications for use with CAD patients.
34. Identify and explain the mechanisms by which exercise may contribute to preventing or rehabilitating individuals with cardiovascular, respiratory, or metabolic diseases.
35. Demonstrate an understanding of the following drug classifications, explain the mechanisms of principle actions, and list the major side effects, including ECG changes at rest and during exercise (see Appendices A and C).
    A. Antianginal (nitrates, beta adrenergic blockers, calcium channel antagonists, etc.)
    B. Antiarrhythmic
    C. Anticoagulant and antiplatelet
    D. Lipid-lowering drugs
    E. Antihypertensive

    F. Digitalis glycosides
    G. Bronchodilators
    H. Hypoglycemics
    I. Psychotropics
    J. Emergency medications
36. Demonstrate an understanding of the various diagnostic and treatment modalities currently used in the management of cardiovascular disease.
37. Describe coronary angiography, radionuclide imaging, echocardiography imaging, and pharmacologic stress studies, including the type of information obtained, sensitivity, specificity, and associated risks and indications for use.
38. Describe PTCA as an alternative to medical management or coronary artery bypass surgery (CABS) in CAD. Demonstrate an understanding of the indications and limitations for PTCA in different subsets of CAD patients vs. CABS or management with medications.
39. Describe the use of thrombolytic therapy in acute MI.

HEALTH APPRAISAL AND FITNESS TESTING

EXERCISE TEST TECHNOLOGIST$_{SM}$

1. Demonstrate the skills and knowledge for administering an exercise test.
2. Recognize inappropriate calibration of testing equipment and explain procedures for calibration, i.e., a motor-driven treadmill, cycle ergometer (mechanical), arm ergometer, electrocardiograph, aneroid and mercury sphygmomanometer, and spirometers.

3. Obtain a routine medical history prior to exercise testing, ensure informed consent is obtained, explain procedures and protocol for the exercise test, recognize the contraindications to an exercise test, and summarize and present screening information to the physician.

4. Recognize the significance of patient medical history and physical exam findings as they relate to exercise testing.

5. Identify patients for whom physician supervision is recommended during maximal and submaximal exercise testing.

6. Perform routine tasks prior to exercise testing including: taking a standard and exercise 12-lead ECG on a participant in the supine, upright, and post-hyperventilation conditions; accurately recording right and left arm blood pressure in different body positions; demonstrating the ability to instruct the test participant in the use of rating of perceived exertion (RPE) scale and other appropriate subjective scales, such as dyspnea and angina scales.

7. Discuss the techniques used to minimize ECG artifact and the value of a single-lead and multiple electrocardiographic lead systems in exercise testing.

8. Discuss the selection of the exercise test protocol in terms of modes of exercise, starting levels, increments of work, length of stages, and frequency of physiologic measures.

9. Discuss how age, weight, level of fitness, and health status are considered in the selection of an exercise test protocol.

10. Contrast exercise testing procedures for pulmonary patients with that of cardiac patients in terms of exercise modality, protocol, physiological measurements, and expected outcomes.

11. Demonstrate appropriate techniques of measurement of physiological and subjective responses, i.e., symptoms, ECG, blood pressure, heart rate, RPE, and O_2 consumption measures at appropriate intervals during the test.

12. Identify appropriate endpoints for exercise testing for various populations.

13. Discuss technical factors that may indicate test termination (e.g., loss of ECG signal, loss of power, etc.).

14. Discuss immediate post-exercise procedures and list various approaches to cool-down.

15. Record, organize, and perform necessary calculations of test data for summary presentation to test interpreter.

16. Describe differences in test protocol and procedures when the exercise involves radionuclide imaging procedures.

17. Demonstrate the ability to administer basic resting spirometric tests including FEV_1, FVC, and MVV.

18. Describe basic equipment and facility requirements for exercise testing.

19. Describe the responsibilities of the exercise test technologist on a typical testing day.

EXERCISE SPECIALIST_{SM}

20. Demonstrate competence in the interpretation of the exercise test for a rehabilitation program.

21. Describe the techniques used to calibrate a motor-driven treadmill, cycle ergometer (mechanical), arm ergometer, electrocardiograph, aneroid and mercury column sphygmomanometer, spirometers, and respiratory gas analyzers.

22. Demonstrate appropriate techniques for measurement of O_2 consumption at appropriate intervals during an exercise test.

23. Modify testing procedures and protocol for children with clinical conditions.

24. Demonstrate the ability to provide objective recommendations to a patient following a cardiovascular event regarding physical conditioning, return to work, and performance of selected activities for daily living (such as driving, stair climbing, sexual activity) based on exercise test results and clinical status.

25. Understand the prognostic implications of the exercise ECG and hemodynamic responses, radionuclide imaging, and holter monitoring in post infarction risk stratification. Use this information in determining the appropriate setting for exercise, level of supervision, and level of monitoring.

ELECTROCARDIOGRAPHY

EXERCISE TEST TECHNOLOGIST_{SM}

1. Demonstrate knowledge of normal and abnormal resting ECGs and be able to recognize commonly encountered abnormalities during exercise testing.

2. Describe the resting ECG by identifying waveforms (P, QRS, T), segments (ST), intervals (PR, QRS, QT), and axis (QRS) which comprise the normal resting ECG.

3. Recognize changes in the ST segment, the presence of abnormal T waves, and significant Q waves as well as their importance in resting and exercise ECGs.

4. Define the ECG criteria for terminating an exercise test due to ischemic changes.

5. Identify ECG patterns of common conduction defects and arrhythmias and their importance at rest and during exercise.

A. Identify ECG changes associated with the following abnormalities:
   1. Bundle branch blocks
   2. Atrioventricular blocks
   3. Sinus bradycardia (<60 beats/min) and tachycardia (>100 beats/min)
   4. Sinus arrest
   5. Supraventricular premature depolarizations and tachycardia
   6. Ventricular premature depolarizations (including frequency, form, couplets, salvos, tachycardia)
   7. Atrial fibrillation
   8. Ventricular fibrillation
B. Define the limits or considerations for initiating and terminating an exercise test based on the ECG abnormalities listed above.

EXERCISE SPECIALIST$_{SM}$

6. Demonstrate an understanding of the important ECG patterns at rest and during exercise in healthy persons and in patients with CAD, pulmonary diseases, ad metabolic diseases.
7. Describe the electrophysiological events involved in the cyclic depolarization and repolarization of the heart.
8. Describe the ECG changes which are associated with myocardial ischemia, injury, and infarction.
   A. Identify ECG complexes typically seen in acute subendocardial ischemia, epicardial injury, and acute and chronic transmural and non Q-wave infarction.
   B. Identify ECG changes which correspond to ischemia in various myocardial regions (inferior,

posterior, anteroseptal, anterior, anterolateral, lateral).

C. Differentiate between Q-wave and non-Q-wave infarction.

9. Identify ECG changes which typically occur due to hyperventilation, electrolyte abnormalities, and drug therapy (see Appendix A).

10. Identify resting ECG changes associated with diseases other than CAD (such as hypertensive heart disease, cardiac chamber enlargement, pericarditis, pulmonary disease, metabolic disorders).

11. Explain possible causes of ischemic ECG changes and various cardiac dysrhythmias. Explain the significance of their occurrence during rest, exercise, and recovery.

12. Identify potentially hazardous dysrhythmias or conduction defects that may be observed on the ECG at rest, during exercise, and recovery. Explain what procedures would be followed in the event of such dysrhythmias or conduction defects.

13. Identify the significance of important ECG abnormalities in the designation of the exercise prescription and in activity selection.

14. Discuss the indications and methods for ECG monitoring during exercise testing and during exercise sessions.

15. Identify ECG patterns with the following conduction defects and dysrhythmias: fascicular blocks and atrial flutter.

PROGRAM DIRECTOR_{SM}

16. Demonstrate the ability to identify ECG patterns and to discuss implications for exercise testing, exercise programming, prognosis, and risk stratification.

17. Explain the diagnostic and prognostic significance of ischemic ECG responses or arrhythmias at rest, during exercise, or recovery.
18. Explain the causes and means of reducing false positive and false negative exercise ECG responses.
19. Understand Baye's theorem as it relates to pretest likelihood of CAD and the predictive value of positive or negative diagnostic exercise ECG results.
20. Discuss the role of ECG exercise testing as it relates to radionuclide imaging and echocardiography imaging.

EMERGENCY PROCEDURES AND SAFETY

EXERCISE TEST TECHNOLOGIST$_{SM}$

1. Demonstrate competency in responding with appropriate emergency procedures to situations which might arise prior to, during, and after administration of an exercise test.
2. List and describe the use of emergency equipment that should be present in an exercise testing laboratory.
3. Demonstrate competency in verifying operating status of and maintaining emergency equipment.
4. Describe emergency procedures for a preventive and rehabilitative exercise testing program.
5. Possess current Basic Cardiac Life Support certification or equivalent credentials, including the use of a pocket airway mask.

EXERCISE SPECIALIST$_{SM}$

6. Demonstrate competence in responding with the appropriate emergency procedures to situations in rehabilitative settings which might arise prior to, during, and after exercise.

7. Describe the emergency response(s) to cardiac arrest, hypoglycemia, bronchospasm, and sudden onset hypotension.
8. Identify the emergency drugs which should be available in exercise testing and participation situations and describe the mechanisms of action.

PROGRAM DIRECTOR$_{SM}$

9. Demonstrate knowledge about appropriate emergency procedures for situations in rehabilitative settings which might arise prior to, during, and after exercise.
10. Diagram an emergency response system and discuss minimum standards for equipment and personnel required in settings for rehabilitative exercise programs.

EXERCISE PROGRAMMING

EXERCISE SPECIALIST$_{SM}$

1. Demonstrate an understanding of the implications of exercise for persons with CAD risk factors and for patients with established cardiovascular, respiratory, metabolic, or orthopedic disorders and demonstrate competence in executing individualized exercise prescription.
2. Discuss the level of supervision and level of monitoring recommended for various patient populations in exercise programs.
3. Prescribe appropriate exercise based on medical information and exercise test data including intensity, duration, frequency, progression, precautions, and type of physical activity.
4. Modify a patient's exercise program (type of physical

activity, intensity, duration, progression) according to the current health status of the patient with the following conditions: immediate post-CABS, MI, PTCA, heart transplantation, COPD, diabetes, obesity, renal disease, and common orthopedic and neuromuscular conditions.

5. Discuss basic mechanisms of action of medications that may affect the exercise prescription: beta adrenergic blockers, diuretics, calcium channel antagonists, antihypertensives, antihistamines, hypoglycemics, tranquilizers, alcohol, diet pills, cold tablets, caffeine, and nicotine.

6. Discuss warm-up and cool-down phenomena with specific reference to angina and ischemic ECG changes, dysrhythmias, and blood pressure changes.

7. Discuss the differences in the physiological responses to arm and leg exercise in cardiac patients.

8. Discuss the appropriate use of static and dynamic exercise by cardiac patients.

9. Design a program of strength training for cardiac patients.

10. Discuss modifications in monitoring of exercise intensity for various patient groups.

11. Discuss possible adverse responses to exercise in various patient groups and what precautions may be taken to prevent them.

12. Discuss contraindications to exercise as related to the current health status of the participant.

13. Given a clinical case study, devise supervised exercise programs for the first 6 weeks after hospitalization for MI, PTCA, CABS, and angina and for the 3 months following.

14. Identify characteristics which correlate or predict poor compliance to exercise programs.

15. Identify and describe the role of various allied health professionals and the indications and procedures for

referral necessary in a multidisciplinary rehabilitation program.

PROGRAM ADMINISTRATION

PROGRAM DIRECTOR_{SM}

1. Demonstrate the ability to administer a clinical program including personnel, finance, program development, and continuous quality improvment.
2. Diagram and explain an organizational chart and show the staff relationships between an exercise program director, governing body, exercise specialist, exercise test technologist, fitness instructor, medical director or advisor, and a participant's personal physician.
3. Identify and explain operating policies for preventive and rehabilitative exercise programs.
4. Describe the role of the medical director and referring physician in the program design and implementation; and describe the responsibility of the program director to these individuals.
5. Describe and explain strategies for enhancing the understanding of the role of rehabilitation on the part of the public, health care policy-makers, health care providers, and the medical community.
6. Discuss the development and implementation of the comprehensive patient care plan.
7. Discuss the role of the rehabilitative staff in the development and implementation of the comprehensive patient care plan.
8. Demonstrate the ability to justify the inclusion of a comprehensive rehabilitation program in the health care setting.

9. Describe the concept of risk stratification and its application to program administration.
10. Identify and explain operating policies for clinical exercise programs including data analysis and reporting, reimbursement of service fees, confidentiality of records, relationships between program and referring physicians, continuing education of participants and family, legal liability, and accident or injury reporting.
11. Demonstrate the ability to assume fiscal (financial) responsibility for clinical programs.
12. Demonstrate the ability to implement and monitor a comprehensive continuous quality improvement process.

INDEX

A

Accupril, 243
Acebutolol, 241
ACSM Certification programs, 299–300
Activity, physical. *See* Physical activity
Adrenalin, 244
Albuterol, 244
Aldactone, 243
Aldomet, 242
Alpha blockers, 241
Altace, 243
Altitude exposure, 294–296
Alupent, 244
American College of Sports Medicine Certifications, 297–306
Amiloride, 243
Amiodarone, 244
Amlodipine, 242
Anthropometric methods, 55–61, 58t, *60–61*
Apresoline, 243
Arrhythmias
    interpretation of test data, 136–140
    supraventricular, 137
    ventricular, 137–140
Artery disease, coronary, graded exercise testing, as screening tool for, 112–123

B

Asthma, interpretation of test data, 147
Atenolol, 241

Benazepril, 243
Benefits, associated with exercise, 3–11
Bepridil, 242
Beta blockers, 241, 244
Betapace, 244
Betaxolal, 241
BIA. *See* Bioelectrical impedance analysis
Bioelectrical impedance analysis, 62–63
Bisoprolol, 241
Blocadren, 241
Blood pressure
    clinical exercise testing, 93, 96–98t
    effect of medication on, 246–252
    exercise testing, 31–32, 33t
    response, interpretation of test data, 129–130, *132,* 133t
Blood profile, exercise testing, 36–37, 37t
Body composition, 53–63
Body fatness, programs for reducing, 217

Brethine, 244
Bretylium, 244
Bretylol, 244
Bronkosol, 244
Bumetanide, 243
Bumex, 243

C

Calan, 242
Calcium channel blockers,
    242, 244
Caloric balance, and
    exercise prescription,
    217–218
Caloric thresholds, for
    adaptation, with exercise
    prescription, 166–167
Capoten, 243
Captopril, 243
Cardene, 242
Cardiac patient
    exercise prescription,
        177–193
    inpatient programs, 98t,
        178–183, 179–181t
    outpatient programs,
        183–189, 184t
        types of, 187–188t,
            187–189
    rate of progression, out-
        patient, 185–186, 186t
    resistance training, 98t,
        189–190, 190t
Cardilate, 242
Cardiorespiratory
    endurance
    exercise prescription,
        156–166
    physical fitness testing,
        63–78

Cardizem, 242
Cardura, 241
Carteolol, 241
Cartrol, 241
Catapres, 242
Children, 220–227
    clinical exercise testing,
        98t, 221–224, 223t
    exercise prescription,
        224–227, 226t
    exercise testing, 220–227
    fitness testing, 220–221,
        221t
Cholesterol, testing,
    exercise, 32–35, 34,
    36t
Cholestyramine, 245
Clinical assessment,
    exercise testing, 29–38
Clinical conditions,
    influencing exercise
    prescription, 206–219
Clinical exercise testing,
    86–109
    blood pressure, 93,
        96–98t
    children, 98t, 221–224,
        223t
    considerations for
        pulmonary patients,
        103–107, 104–105t
    electrocardiographic
        (ECG) monitoring,
        97–99
    exercise protocols,
        92–93, 94
    exercise test modalities,
        91–92
    expired gases, 93–97
    heart rate, 93, 96–98t

Clinical exercise testing
(continued)
 heart rate and blood
  pressure, 93, 96–98t
 indications
  and applications,
   86–91, *88–90*
  for exercise test
   termination, 98t, 101
 lung function, 105
 measurements, 93–100
 methodology, 107
 non-exercise stress tests
  or pharmacological
  tests, 102–103
 post-exercise period,
  100–101
 pulmonary patients,
  103–107
 radionuclide exercise
  testing, 102
 subjective ratings,
  99–100
Clinical test data, interpretation of, 130–140
Clinical Track, 302–304
 Certification KSAs,
  335–354
Clonidine, 242
Cold temperature, 294
Colestid, 245
Colestipol, 245
Common field test
 equations, 284
Common medications,
 241–252
Composition, body, 53–63
Conditioning stage, initial,
 with exercise
 prescription, 169

Continuous positive airway
 pressure (CPAP),
 pulmonary patients, 201
Continuous protocols, *vs.*
 discontinuous
 (intermittent), in
 physical fitness testing,
 66–67
Contraindications, to
 exercise testing, 38–41,
 42t
COPD, interpretation of
 test data, 147
Cordarone, 244
Corgard, 241
Coronary artery disease,
 graded exercise testing,
 as screening tool for,
 112–123
Coumadin, 245
CPAP. *See* Continuous
 positive airway pressure
 (CPAP)
Cromolyn sodium, 244

D

Data
 integration of, in exercise
  prescription, 162–163
 interpretation, 110–150
  arrhythmias, 136–140
  asthma, 147
  blood pressure
   response, 129–130,
   132, 133t
  clinical test data,
   130–140
  COPD, 147
  ECG waveforms,
   133–134

Data *(continued)*
  exercise capacity,
    88–89, 124–128
  exercise testing,
    comparison with
    radionuclide
    imaging, 145
  fitness test, 110–111,
    111–128t
  graded exercise
    testing, screening
    tool, coronary artery
    disease, 112–123
  heart rate response,
    128–129, *131–132*
  interpretation of
    exercise tests in
    pulmonary patients,
    146
  interstitial lung
    disease, 147
  predictive value of
    exercise testing,
    140t, 140–148
  prognostic
    applications of the
    exercise test,
    145–146
  psychogenic dyspnea,
    147
  pulmonary vascular
    disease, 147
  of responses to graded
    exercise testing,
    124–130
  sensitivity, 141t,
    141–142
  specific respiratory
    diseases, 147–148
    specificity, 142t,
      142–143
    ST segment changes,
      134–136, *138*
    supraventricular
      arrhythmias, 137
    symptom limitation,
      147–148
    value, 143–144, 144t
    ventricular
      arrhythmias,
      137–140
Diabetes mellitus, exercise
  prescription, 210–212t,
  213–215
Digoxin, 242
Diltiazem, 242
Diltrate, 242
Dipyridamole, 245
Direct calorimetry, 269–270
Discontinuous
  (intermittent), *vs.*
  continuous protocols, in
  physical fitness testing,
  66–67
Disopyramide, 244
Doxazosin, 241
Duration, in exercise
  prescription, 163
  for pulmonary patients,
  199
Dyazide, 243
DynaCirc, 242
Dyrenium, 243
Dyspnea, psychogenic, 147

E
ECG interpretation,
  263–268, 264

ECG monitoring. *See* Electrocardiographic monitoring

ECG waveforms, interpretation of test data, 133–134

Edecrin, 243

Elderly
exercise prescription, 228–235
exercise testing, 98t, 228–235, 230t
flexibility, 234–235
resistance training, 231–233

Electrocardiography, 347–350
clinical exercise testing, 97–99

Electrode placement, precordial (chest) leads, 263

Emergency equipment, and drugs, 254

Emergency management, 253–262

Emergency procedures/safety, 321–323, 350 351

Enalapril, 243

Encainide, 244

Endurance, cardiorespiratory, exercise prescription, 156–166

Enkaid, 244

Environment
considerations, 288–296
with physical fitness testing, 52

Ephedrine, 244

Epinephrine, 244

Ergometer tests, submaximal cycle, physical fitness testing, 68–71, *69,* 70t, *72*

Esidrix, 243

Estimation of energy expenditure—metabolic calculations, 273–275

Ethacrynic acid, 243

Ethmozine, 244

Evaluation, pre-test, 29–48

Exercise
benefits associated with, 3–11
capacity, data, interpretation, *88–89,* 124–128
duration, in exercise prescription, 163
frequency, with exercise prescription, 163–166
intensity, exercise prescription, 158–163
physiology, 309–312, 330–337
policies, and safety, 9–10
programming, 323–327, 351–353
protocol, clinical exercise testing, 92–93, *94*
public health perspective, 3
risks of, 3–11
testing, pre-test evaluation, 29–48

Exercise prescription,
    151–240
  art of, 155–156
  caloric balance, 217–218
  caloric thresholds for
    adaptation, 166–167
  cardiac patient
    inpatient programs,
      98t, 178–183,
      179–181t
    outpatient programs,
      183–189, 184t
      types of, 187–188t,
      187–189
    outpatient rate of
      progression,
      185–186, 186t
    resistance training,
      98t, 189–190, 190t
  cardiorespiratory
    endurance, 156–166
  children, 224–227, 226t
  clinical conditions
    influencing, 206–219
  diabetes mellitus,
    210–212t, 213–215
  elderly, 228–235
  exercise duration, 163
  exercise frequency,
    163–166
  fatness, programs for
    reducing, 217
  general principles of,
    153–176
  heart rate, 159–160, *161,*
    162t
  hypertension, 33t,
    206–209, 210–212t
  improvement stage,
    169–170

initial conditioning
    stage, 169
integration of data,
    162–163
intensity, of exercise,
    158–163
maintenance stage, 170
METs, 157t, 162,
    164–165t
mode of exercise,
    156–158, 157t
muscular fitness,
    172–174
musculoskeletal
    flexibility, 170–171
obesity, 210–212t,
    216–219
peripheral vascular
    disease, 209–213,
    210–212t
program supervision,
    175t, 175–176
pulmonary patients,
    194–199
  alternative modes of
    exercise training,
    201–202
  continuous positive
    airway pressure
    (CPAP), 201
  duration, 199
  frequency, 195
  intensity, 195–199,
    196–197t
  mode of exercise, 195
  program design and
    supervision,
    203–204
  pursed-lips breathing,
    199–200

Exercise prescription
(continued)
  pulmonary patients
    (continued)
    resistive inspiratory
      muscle training
      (RIMT), 202, 203t
    supplemental oxygen,
      200–201
    upper body resistance
      training, 201–202
  purposes of, 154–155
  rate of progression,
    167–170, 168t
  RPE scales, 160–162, 162t
  and weight loss
    programs, 218–219
Exercise testing, 27–150
  blood pressure, 31–32, 33t
  blood profile, 36–37, 37t
  children, 220–227
  cholesterol, 32–35, *34,*
    36t
  clinical exercise testing,
    86–109
    blood pressure, 93,
      96–98t
    electrocardiographic
      (ECG) monitoring,
      97–99
    exercise protocols,
      92–93, *94*
    exercise test
      modalities, 91–92
    expired gases, 93–97
    heart rate and blood
      pressure, 93, 96–98t
    indications and
      applications, 86–91,
      88–90
  indications for
    exercise test
    termination, 98t, 101
  lung function, 105
  measurements, 93–100
  methodology, 107
  non-exercise stress
    test, 102–103
  post-exercise period,
    100–101
  pulmonary patients,
    103–107, 104–105t
  radionuclide exercise
    testing, 102
  subjective ratings,
    99–100
comparison with
  radionuclide imaging,
  145
contraindications to,
  38–41, 42t
elderly, 98t, 228–229,
  230t
laboratory tests, 25t,
  29–31, 30–32t
lipoproteins and, 32–35,
  34, 36t
medical history, 25t,
  29–31, 30–32t
patient instructions,
  47–48
physical examination,
  25t, 29–31, 30–32t
physical fitness
  guidelines, 51–52
  purposes of, 50–51
physical fitness testing
  anthropometric
  methods, 55–61, 58t,
  60–61

Exercise testing *(continued)*
  physical fitness testing
    (continued)
    bioelectrical
      impedance analysis,
      62–63
    body composition,
      53–63
    cardiorespiratory
      endurance, 63–78
    discontinuous
      (intermittent) *vs.*
      continuous
      protocols, 66–67
    field tests, 73–75
    flexibility, 83–84, 84t
    hydrostatic weighing,
      53–54
    infrared interactance,
      62–63
    maximal *vs.*
      submaximal exercise
      testing, 64–66, *65*
    mode of testing, 68–75
    muscular endurance,
      81–82, 82t
    muscular fitness, 78–84
    muscular strength,
      80–81
    pretest instructions, 51
    skinfold
      measurements, 55,
      56–57t
    step tests, 73
    subjective rating
      scales, use of, 67–68,
      68t
    submaximal cycle
      ergometer tests,
      68–71, *69,* 70t, *72*
    submaximal treadmill
      tests, 71–73, *74*
    test environment, 52
    test order, 52
    test sequence and
      measures, 75–77
    test termination
      criteria, 77, 78t
    $\dot{V}O_2$max, 63–64
  predictive value of, 140t,
    140–148
  pregnancy, 235–239,
    236–238t
  prognostic applications
    of, 145–146
  pulmonary function,
    37–38, 39–40t
  pulmonary patients,
    interpretation of, 146
  risks associated with,
    6–8
Expired gases, clinical
  exercise testing, 93–97

F
Fatness, programs for
  reducing, 217
Felodipine, 242
Field test
  equations, 283–284
  physical fitness testing,
    73–75
Fitness
  muscular, with exercise
    prescription, 172–174
  test, 110–111, 111–128t.
    See Physcial fitness
    testing
    children, 220–221, 221t

Fitness *(continued)*
  test, *(continued)*
    data, interpretation of,
      110–111, 111–128t
Flecainide, 244
Flexibility
  elderly, 234–235
  musculoskeletal,
    exercise prescription,
    170–171
  in physical fitness
    testing, 83–84, 84t
Fluvastatin, 245
Formulas for estimating
  maximal and target heart
  rates, 274
Fosinopril, 243
Frequency of exercise, with
  exercise prescription,
  163–166
Functional anatomy and
  biomechanics, 307–308,
  335–336
Furosemide, 243

G

Gamfibrozil, 245
Gases, expired, clinical
  exercise testing, 93–97
Generic/brand names, of
  common drugs, by class,
  241–245
Graded exercise testing, as
  screening tool, for
  coronary artery disease,
  112–123
Guanabenz, 242
Guanadrel, 242
Guanethidine, 242
Guanfacine, 242

H

Health/Fitness Track,
  300–302
Health appraisal/fitness
  testing, 318–321,
  344–347
Health promotion, 334
Health screening
  for physical activity,
    12–13, *14,* 17–18t
  and risk stratification,
    12–25
Health/Fitness Track,
  Certification KSAs,
  307–334
Heart rate
  clinical exercise testing,
    93, 96–98t
  effect of medication on,
    246–252
  exercise prescription,
    159–160, *161,* 162t
  response, interpretation
    of data, 128–129,
    131–132
Heat/humidity, effect of,
  288–293
HR. *See* Heart rate
Human
  behavior/psychology,
    317–318, 338–339
Human
  development/aging,
    312–313, 338
Hydralazine, 243
Hydrochlorothiazide
  (HCTZ), 243
Hydrostatic weighing,
  53–54
Hylorel, 242

Hypertension, exercise
     prescription, 33t,
     206–209, 210–212t
Hytrin, 241

I

Imaging, radionuclide,
     comparison with
     exercise testing, 145
Improvement stage,
     exercise prescription,
     169–170
Inderal, 241
Indirect calorimetry,
     270–271
Informed consent, 41–47
Infrared interactance,
     62–63
Initial conditioning stage,
     with exercise
     prescription, 169
Inpatient programs, cardiac
     patient, 98t, 178–183,
     179–181t
Inspiratory muscle
     training, resistive,
     pulmonary patients, 202,
     203t
Instructions, to patient,
     with exercise testing,
     47–48
Intal, 244
Integration of data, in
     exercise prescription,
     162–163
Intensity
     of exercise, exercise
          prescription, 158–163
     for pulmonary patients,
          195–199, 196–197t

Interpretation of test data,
     110–150
     arrhythmias, 136–140
     asthma, 147
     blood pressure response,
          129–130, *132*, 133t
     clinical test data,
          130–140
     COPD, 147
     ECG waveforms,
          133–134
     exercise capacity, *88–89*,
          124–128
     exercise testing,
          comparison with
          radionuclide imaging,
          145
     graded exercise testing as
          a screening tool for
          coronary artery
          disease, 112–123
     heart rate response,
          128–129, *131–132*
     interpretation, of
          responses to graded
          exercise testing,
          124–130
     interstitial lung disease,
          147
     predictive value of
          exercise testing, 140t,
          140–148
     prognostic applications
          of the exercise test,
          145–146
     psychogenic dyspnea,
          147
     pulmonary disease, 147
     sensitivity, 141t, 141–142
     specificity, 142t, 142–143

Interpretation of test data
  (continued)
  ST segment changes,
    134–136, *138*
  supraventricular
    arrhythmias, 137
  symptom limitation,
    147–148
  ventricular arrhythmias,
    137–140
Interstitial lung disease,
  interpretation of test
  data, 147
Ismelin, 242
Ismo, 242
Isoetharine, 244
Isordil, 242
Isosorbide dinitrate, 242
Isosorbide mononitrate, 242
Isradipine, 242

K

Kerlone, 241
Knowledge, Skills, and
  Abilities (KSAs)
  underlying ACSM
  Certifications, 304–306

L

Labetalol, 242
Laboratory tests, and
  exercise testing, 25t,
  29–31, 30–32t
Lanoxin, 242
Lasix, 243
Lescol, 245
Levatol, 241
Lidocaine, 244

Life-threatening situation,
  plan for, 257–259,
  260–262
Lipoproteins, and exercise
  testing, 32–35, *34,* 36t
Lisinopril, 243
Localizing and naming
  transmural infarcts, 266
Loniten, 243
Loop diuretic, 243
Lopid, 245
Lopressor, 241
Lorelco, 245
Lotensin, 243
Lovastatin, 245
Lung
  disease, interstitial,
    interpretation of test
    data, 147
  function, clinical
    exercise testing, 105

M

Maintenance stage,
  exercise prescription,
  170
Maximal, *vs.* submaximal
  exercise testing, 64–66,
  65
Measurement
  clinical exercise testing,
    93–100
  skinfold, 55, 56–57t
  of VO_2, 271–272
Measurement and
  estimation of energy
  expenditure, 269–287
Medical history, prior to
  exercise testing, 25t,
  29–31, 30–32t

Metaproterenol, 244
Methyldopa, 242
Metolazone, 243
Metoprolol, 241
METs, 157t, 162, 164–165t
Mevacor, 245
Mexiletine, 244
Mexitil, 244
Midamor, 243
Minipress, 241
Minoxidil, 243
Moduretic, 243
Monopril, 243
Moricizine, 244
Muscular fitness,
    exercise prescription,
    172–174
    physical fitness testing,
    78–84, 82t
Muscular strength, 80–81
Musculoskeletal flexibility,
    170–171

N

Nadolol, 241
Nicardipine, 242
Nicobid, 245
Nicotinic acid (niacin), 245
Nifedipine, 242
Nimodipine, 242
Nimotop, 242
Nitroglycerin, 242
    ointment, 242
    patches, 242
Nitrol ointment, 242
Nitrostat, 242
Nonemergency situations,
    plan for, 255–256

Normal values for the QT
    interval as a function of
    heart rate, 266
Norpace, 244
Norvasc, 242
Nutrition and weight
    management, 327–329

O

Obesity, exercise
    prescription, 210–212t,
    216–219
Order of tests, physical
    fitness testing, 52
Outpatient program
    cardiac patient, 183–189,
        184t
        types of, 187–188t,
        187–189
    rate of progression,
        cardiac patient,
        185–186, 186t
Oxygen, supplemental, for
    pulmonary patients,
    200–201

P

Pathophysiology/risk
    factors, 313–316,
    340–344
Patient instructions, with
    exercise testing, 47–48
Penbutolol, 241
Pentaerythritol tetranitrate,
    242
Pentoxifylline, 245

Peripheral vascular
  disease, exercise
  prescription, 209–213,
  210–212t
Persantine, 245
Pharmacological tests,
  non-exercise, 102–103
Physical activity. *See also*
  Exercise
  health screening for,
    12–13, *14,* 17–18t
  regular, benefits of, 4–6,
    5–6t
  risks associated with,
    8–10
Physical examination, and
  exercise testing, 25t,
  29–31, 30–32t
Physical fitness testing,
  49–85
  anthropometric methods,
    55–61, 58t, *60–61*
  basic principles, 51–52
  bioelectrical impedance
    analysis, 62–63
  body composition, 53–63
  cardiorespiratory
    endurance, 63–78
  discontinuous
    (intermittent) *vs.*
    continuous protocols,
    66–67
  field tests, 73–75
  flexibility, 83–84, 84t
  guidelines, 51–52
  hydrostatic weighing,
    53–54
  infrared interactance,
    62–63

maximal *vs.* submaximal
    exercise testing, 64–66,
    65
  mode of testing, 68–75
  muscular endurance,
    81–82, 82t
  muscular fitness, 78–84
  muscular strength, 80–81
  pretest instructions, 51
  purposes of, 50–51
  skinfold measurements,
    55, 56–57t
  step tests, 73
  subjective rating scales,
    use of, 67–68, 68t
  submaximal cycle
    ergometer tests, 68–71,
    69, 70t, *72*
  submaximal treadmill
    tests, 71–73, *74*
  test environment, 52
  test order, 52
  test sequence and
    measures, 75–77
  test termination criteria,
    77, 78t
  VO$_2$max, 63–64
Pindolol, 241
Plendil, 242
Policy, exercise, and safety,
  9–10
Post-exercise period,
  clinical exercise testing,
  100–101
Potassium-sparing, 243
Practice metabolic
  calculations (with
  answers), 286–287
Pravachol, 245

Pravastatin, 245
Prazosin, 241
Precordial (chest) lead electrode placement, 263
Predictive value, of exercise testing, 140t, 140–148
Pregnancy, exercise, 235–239, 236–238t
Prescription, exercise, 151–240
  art of, 155–156
  caloric balance, 217–218
  caloric thresholds for adaptation, 166–167
  cardiac patient, 177–193
    inpatient programs, 98t, 178–183, 179–181t
    outpatient programs, 183–189, 184t
      types of, 187–188t, 187–189
    resistance training, 98t, 189–190, 190t
  cardiorespiratory endurance, 156–166
  children, 224–227, 226t
  clinical conditions influencing, 206–219
  diabetes mellitus, 210–212t, 213–215
  elderly, 228–235
  exercise duration, 163
  exercise frequency, 163–166
  fatness, programs for reducing, 217
  general principles of, 153–176

  heart rate, 159–160, *161,* 162t
  hypertension, 33t, 206–209, 210–212t
  improvement stage, 169–170
  initial conditioning stage, 169
  integration of data, 162–163
  intensity, of exercise, 158–163
  maintenance stage, 170
  METs, 157t, 162, 164–165t
  mode of exercise, 156–158, 157t
  muscular fitness, 172–174
  musculoskeletal flexibility, 170–171
  obesity, 210–212t, 216–219
  peripheral vascular disease, 209–213, 210–212t
  program supervision, 175t, 175–176
  pulmonary patients, 194–205
    alternative modes of exercise training, 201–202
    continuous positive airway pressure (CPAP), 201
    duration, 199
    frequency, 195
    intensity, 195–199, 196–197t

Prescription, exercise
(continued)
  pulmonary patients
    (continued)
    mode of exercise, 195
    program design and
      supervision,
      203–204
    pursed-lips breathing,
      199–200
    resistive inspiratory
      muscle training
      (RIMT), 202, 203t
    supplemental oxygen,
      200–201
    upper body resistance
      training, 201–202
  purposes of, 154–155
  rate of progression,
    167–170, 168t
  RPE scales, 160–162, 162t
  and weight loss
    programs, 218–219
Pretest instructions, with
  physical fitness testing,
  51
Prinivil, 243
Probucol, 245
Procainamide, 244
Procardia, 242
Prognostic applications, of
  exercise test, 145–146
Program administration,
  329–333, 353–354
Program supervision,
  exercise prescription,
  175t, 175–176
Progression, rate of, with
  exercise prescription,
  167–170, 168t

Pronestyl, 244
Propranolol, 241
Protocols, clinical exercise
  testing, 92–93, *94*
Proventil, 244
Psychogenic dyspnea,
  interpretation of test
  data, 147
Public health perspective,
  exercise, 3
Pulmonary function
  testing, 37–38, 39–40t
Pulmonary patients
  alternative modes of
    exercise training,
    201–202
  clinical exercise testing,
    105–107
  considerations for, in
    clinical exercise
    testing, 103–107,
    104–105t
  continuous positive
    airway pressure
    (CPAP), 201
  duration of exercise for,
    199
  exercise prescription,
    194–205
  frequency of exercise for,
    195
  intensity of exercise for,
    195–199, 196–197t
  interpretation of exercise
    tests, 146
  mode of exercise, 195
  program design and
    supervision, 203–204
  pursed-lips breathing,
    199–200

Pulmonary patients
(continued)
resistive inspiratory
muscle training
(RIMT), 202, 203t
supplemental oxygen,
200–201
upper body resistance
training, 201–202
Pulmonary vascular
disease, interpretation of
test data, 147
Pursed-lips breathing,
pulmonary patients,
199–200

Q
Questran, 245
Quinapril, 243
Quinidex, 244
Quinidine, 244

R
Radionuclide exercise
testing, 102
Radionuclide imaging,
comparison with
exercise testing, 145
Ramipril, 243
Rate, of heart, prescription,
exercise, 159–160, *161,*
162t
Reserpine, 242
Resistance training
cardiac patient, 98t,
189–190, 190t
elderly, 231–233
upper body, pulmonary
patients, 201–202

Resistive inspiratory
muscle training (RIMT),
pulmonary patients, 202,
203t
Respiratory diseases,
interpretation of test
data, 147–148
Respiratory exchange ratio
(R) and respiratory
quotient (RQ), 272–273
RIMT. *See* Resistive
inspiratory muscle
training (RIMT)
Risk
associated with exercise,
3–11
of exercise testing, 6–8
with physical activity,
8–10
stratification of, 13–19,
19–25t
and health screening,
12–25
RPE scales, with exercise
prescription, 160–162,
162t

S
Safety, and exercise policy,
9–10
Screening
for physical activity,
12–13, *14,* 17–18t
and risk stratification,
12–25
for coronary artery
disease, graded
exercise testing,
112–123

Sectral, 241
Sensitivity of test data,
141t, 141–142
Serapasil, 242
Serum enzymes
(myocardial tissue
necrosis), 268
Simvastatin, 245
Skinfold measurements,
55, 56–57t
Sotalol, 244
Specificity, of test data,
142t, 142–143
Spironolactone, 243
ST segment changes,
interpretation of test
data, 134–136, *138*
Step tests, physical fitness
testing, 73
Stepwise approach to using
metabolic calculations,
275–283
Stress tests,
pharmacological or non-
exercise, 102–103
Subjective rating
in clinical exercise
testing, 99–100
in physical fitness
testing, 67–68, 68t
Submaximal, *vs.* maximal
exercise testing, 64–66, *65*
Submaximal cycle
ergometer tests, 68–71,
69, 70t, *72*
Submaximal treadmill
tests, 71–73, *74*
Supervision
of program, with exercise
prescription, 175t,
175–176
pulmonary patients,
203–204
Supplemental oxygen,
pulmonary patients,
200–201
Supraventricular
arrhythmias, 137
Supraventricular *vs.*
ventricular ectopic beats,
267
Symptom limitation,
interpretation of test
data, 147–148

T

Tambocor, 244
Tenex, 242
Tenormin, 241
Terazosin, 241
Termination, indications
for, clinical exercise
testing, 98t, 101
Test data, interpretation of,
110–150
arrhythmias, 136–140
asthma, 147
blood pressure response,
129–130, *132,* 133t
clinical test data,
130–140
COPD, 147
ECG waveforms, 133–
134
exercise capacity, *88–89,*
124–128

Test data, interpretation of, (continued)
  exercise testing, comparison with radionuclide imaging, 145
  graded exercise testing, as screening tool, coronary artery disease, 112–123
  heart rate response, 128–129, *131–132*
  interpretation
    exercise tests in pulmonary patients, 146
    responses, to graded exercise testing, 124–130
  interstitial lung disease, 147
  predictive value of exercise testing, 140t, 140–148
  prognostic applications of the exercise test, 145–146
  psychogenic dyspnea, 147
  pulmonary vascular disease, 147
  sensitivity, 141t, 141–142
  specificity, 142t, 142–143
  ST segment changes, 134–136, *138*
  supraventricular arrhythmias, 137
  symptom limitation, 147–148
  ventricular arrhythmias, 137–140
Test environment, with physical fitness testing, 52
Test order, with physical fitness testing, 52
Test sequence and measures, physical fitness testing, 75–77
Test termination criteria, physical fitness testing, 77, 78t
Testing, exercise, 27–150
  blood pressure, 31–32, 33t
  blood profile analyses, 36–37, 37t
  cholesterol, 32–35, *34, 36t*
  clinical assessment, 29–38
  contraindications to, 38–41, 42t
  laboratory tests, 25t, 29–31, 30–32t
  lipoproteins and, 32–35, *34,* 36t
  medical history, 25t, 29–31, 30–32t
  patient instructions, 47–48
  physical examination, 25t, 29–31, 30–32t
  pre-test evaluation, 29–48
  pulmonary function, 37–38, 39–40t
  risks, 6–8
Thiazides, 242

Timolol, 241
Tocainide, 244
Tonocard, 244
Trandate, 242
Transderm Nitro, 242
Trental, 245
Triamterene, 243

U

Upper body resistance
 training, pulmonary
 patients, 201–202

V

Value of exercise test data,
 143–144, 144t
Vascor, 242
Vascular disease,
 peripheral, exercise
  prescription, 209–213,
  210–212t
 pulmonary,
  interpretation of test
  data, 147
Vasotec, 243
Ventricular arrhythmias,
 137–140

Verapamil, 242
Visken, 241
VO$_2$max, physical fitness
 testing, 63–64

W

Warfarin, 245
Waveforms, ECG,
 interpretation of test
 data, 133–134
Weighing, hydrostatic,
 53–54
Weight loss programs, and
 exercise prescription,
 218–219
Wyntensin, 242

X

Xylocaine, 244

Z

Zaroxolyn, 243
Zebeta, 241
Zestril, 243
Zocor, 245